The Looming Epidemic

The Impact of HIV and AIDS in India

The Looming Epidemic

The Impact of HIV and AIDS in India

Edited by
PETER GODWIN

HURST & COMPANY
London

Published in the United Kingdom by
C. Hurst & Co. (Publishers) Ltd.
38 King Street, London WC2E 8JZ

1-85065-424-7

Published by arrangement with
Mosaic Books, New Delhi 110024, India.

Printed in India

Contents

Foreword

The past half century since the end of the second world war has witnessed truly revolutionary changes in mortality or the average length of human life, particularly in the developing countries. The average number of years lived by a person on planet earth has risen from 46.5 during 1950–55 to 64.3 during 1990–95 in the world as a whole and from 40.9 to 62.1 in the developing world.

Unfortunately, the welcome changes achieved so far through the control of infectious and parasitic diseases are now threatened by the reported growing resistance of the vectors of malaria and other microbes to the widely used antibiotics and other drugs. There is widespread fear also of the emergence of some new pathogens or diseases, not present on the planet so far, which can cause considerable morbidity and mortality.

The scientific thinking on these issues has been stimulated partly by the emergence in the early 1980s of the new dreaded disease, HIV/AIDS (Human Immunodeficiency Virus, which causes the Acquired Immuno Deficiency Syndrome), which was first identified around 1983 both in the USA and in Africa. The United Nations AIDS Organisation has estimated that at the end of 1996, about 23 million persons were infected with AIDS, and more than six million had already died because of AIDS. The number of HIV-infected persons in India is currently placed at between 3 to 5 million, and it is widely feared that it might assume epidemic proportions, at least in some states of the country. There is considerable controversy about these numbers, as well as the magnitude of impact, especially at the macro level. However, if in fact India currently has several million infected individuals, there is little doubt that in the country as a whole, the number of cases will be large enough to pose a severe crisis for very many households. Further, since cases will be scattered throughout the length and breadth of our continental country, prevention and impact alleviation will pose a major challenge for the policymakers.

The HIV/AIDS epidemic will certainly raise both the private and the public sector costs of health in the country. Some of these costs will be a consequence of the increased general morbidity (particularly TB, pneumonia, gastroenteritis, hepatitis, etc.) because of the impaired immune systems of large numbers of people. Evidence suggests that the expenditures by HIV patients seeking 'cure' as well as getting treated for opportunistic infections from different sources (including quacks and alternative systems of medicine) are quite high. In fact, many of the patients and their families will not associate the illnesses and the death with HIV or AIDS even after getting the diagnosis. Some other aspects of the household level impact of the epidemic will result from high treatment costs including reduced resource allocation to essential consumption, reduced nutrition of especially mothers and children, reduced savings and liquidation of assets, etc.

In addition to the household spending on medical and drug bills, there will be systems costs of prevention, as well as higher costs of health care due to increased demand. There is also the danger of reduced supply of health care for other non-AIDS diseases due to this increased demand, which would further raise the costs of health care across the board.

One final aspect of the HIV/AIDS epidemic is the high level of discrimination which results from lack of awareness and ignorance about the infection and the modes of its transmission and prevention. In India there have been many instances of discrimination and stigmatisation including bizarre mob behaviour.

It is clear that the epidemic will ultimately affect many more sectors of the economy and different sections of the society. Given this perspective, it is high time that we establish a comprehensive research agenda on various issues relating to health as well as specifically to HIV/AIDS, and mobilise the requisite human and financial resources for the purpose. Both quantitative and qualitative research is urgently necessary and the relevant training efforts need to be expanded. A research agenda with respect to AIDS must include, as this book shows, the following issues:

• the magnitude of changes in morbidity patterns resulting from the spread of HIV in India;

• the costs of public and private health care likely to be associated with these changes;

• alternative mechanisms through which these costs might be met;

• effects of significant changes in young adult mortality rates on the economic and social system;

• the likely distribution of these changes around the country;

• costs of responding to these changes;

• the costs and benefits associated with different HIV-related policy options, such as provision of anti-retroviral therapies, AZT for pregnant women, different approaches to terminal care, etc.

As the book suggests, data and quantitative assessments are urgently needed on all these issues. The book also suggests some of the techniques and approaches necessary for such assessments.

Over the past five years, the Institute of Economic Growth (IEG) has already addressed some aspects of the research agenda outlined here. One of the earliest studies of the economic impact of HIV in Asia was conducted at IEG in 1994; and one of the chapters in this book has been written by a colleague at the IEG. The IEG is continuing this effort by undertaking more research on varied aspects of health, including AIDS. I am very happy, therefore, to write this Foreword, and to support the policy-oriented research agenda advocated by this book. I trust this book will stimulate adequate response from the community of researchers and policy-makers interested in the health of the Indian people.

Pravin Visaria
Director, IEG
Delhi 110 007

June 1998

A Note about the Authors

DR SHAHID ASHRAF is an economist specialising in health and labour. A gold medallist from Aligarh Muslim University where he got his MA degree, he obtained his MPhil from Jawaharlal Nehru University and his PhD in Economics from Punjab University. He taught at Aligarh Muslim University from 1983 to 1986 and is presently at Jamia Milia University. He has worked as a consultant to the International Labour Organisation, primarily on child labour in India, UNDP, the Family Planning Association of India, and other organisations. He has authored two books, most recently a textbook on computational methods for undergraduates, and a number of reports and articles.

DR TONY BARNETT is Professor of Development Studies at the School of Development Studies, University of East Anglia. He got his BA from the University of Hull in Sociology, Politics, Social Anthropology and Economics, and his MA and PhD in Economics from the University of Manchester. He was previously Lecturer in Sociology of the Middle East at the University of Durham in the UK. He has been adviser and consultant to many multilateral agencies, and governments and NGOs; was previously a trustee of Oxfam UK and Ireland; and has spent almost thirty years of research and other work on social and economic change in Africa, South East Asia, the Pacific, the Middle East and India. He is currently also Overseas Visiting Professor at the Institute of Developing Economics Advanced School, Tokyo, Japan. He has been researching the social and economic impact of HIV/AIDS since 1986, and is co-author, with Piers Blaikie, of the seminal book *AIDS in Africa*.

DR S.C. CHAWLA has for the last five years been Professor and Head of the Department of Social and Preventive Medicine at the Lady Hardinge Medical College in New Delhi, where he has been responsible for a number of studies on HIV and AIDS, as well as many orientation and training courses on the issue for medical practitioners, faculty and postgraduate students. In more than thirty-three years of professional life he has worked in the Maulana Azad Medical College, on the smallpox eradication campaign, in Asia's largest TB hospital, as consultant, trainer, and co-ordinator for a number of national public health issues, and as a member of the Planning Group for the National Immunisation Programme; all in additon to his 15 years with the Lady Hardinge Medical College.

EMMANUEL ELIOT is a French geographer and reader in the Human Sciences Department of the University of Le Havre and Rouen in Normandy, specialising in health geography, health systems and diseases. His Masters/M Phil degree dealt with health care supply within the middle classes in Coimbatore. Tamil Nadu. He is currently completing a PhD on HIV diffusion in India, particularly Mumbai and Andhra Pradesh, and working with a variety of GIS systems to examine the spatial distribution and spread patterns of HIV.

PETER GODWIN has been associated professionally and personally with India since 1977, when he came to the UNICEF in New Delhi, and married here, having previously been with the WHO in Indonesia and Sri Lanka. He then spent five years with AMREF in East Africa, and six with the Population Welfare Division and the National Institute of Health in Islamabad. He has worked for the last six years on the HIV epidemic, in Kenya with the World Bank, and in Asia, where he was for three years the Chief of the UNDP Regional HIV Project for Asia and the Pacific. Though a historian by study and an educationist by training, he has worked in the fields of health, population, nutrition and development for nearly thirty years and in more than twelve countries. He has recently had two books published on HIV and AIDS: *The Economics of HIV and AIDS: the Case of South and South East Asia* which he edited with David Bloom, for Oxford University Press, New Delhi, and *The Socio-economic Implications of the Epidemic*, published by UNDP, New Delhi. He is currently the HIV/AIDS Adviser to the Royal Government of Cambodia.

DR INDRANI GUPTA is an economist presently affiliated to the Institute of Economic Growth at Delhi University. She completed her PhD from the University of Maryland in labour economics, and her current research interests include labour. health and development economics. She began her career as an economist with the Government of India, and after getting her PhD, joined the Policy Research Department of the World Bank, where she worked on the Kagera Project, a household-based survey of the economic impact of fatal adult illness, from AIDS and other causes, in Tanzania. Since her return to India in 1994, she has continued to work on HIV/AIDS in addition to her other research interests. Her chapter in this book is one example of her continued dedication to find ways to alleviate the impact of the epidemic.

SWATI GUPTA is a public health specialist at the New York City Health Department. During her public health training at Yale in 1996, she did a field internship at the ARCON Centre in Mumbai. As part of her internship, she conducted a study of the knowledge, attitudes and practice regarding HIV/AIDS, including the perceived impact of the epidemic, at seven large industries in Mumbai. She is presently monitoring the epidemic of tuberculosis in the New York Council District.

Dr Subash **Hira** is an Indian physician who specialised in sexually transmitted diseases, infectious diseases and public health. He worked in Zambia as the Director of the National STD/AIDS Control Programme for over a decade, witnessing and extensively documenting the emergence of the HIV/AIDS epidemic in Central Africa, and its subsequent course and impact. He carries with him the rich experience of designing training and intervention programmes at national and international levels, and continues to be closely associated with research, training, interventions, country programme designing, implementation, and evaluation studies. Presently, he is Director of the AIDS Research and Control Centre (ARCON) in Mumbai, a collaborative programme of the Government of Maharashtra and the University of Texas, Houston. He is also, under the World Bank assistance to the Government of India, Technical Advisor to the National AIDS Control Organisation (NACO).

Dr Indira **Koithra** graduated from the London School Economics, received her PhD from the University of Singapore. She is at present Chairman of 'Gleneagles', Singapore and India, and Director of the Vishwa Yuvak Kendra (International Youth Centre), New Delhi India, Vice President of OISCA International (India), and President of the Women's World Summit Foundation (Singapore). She has worked for the last twenty years, as a scholar and in public life, for the advancement of women and youth. She has participated in and contributed to numerous seminars and conferences in over twenty countries and to several publications and journals; she was the editor of "Women Studies and Women in Development: bridging the gap", and has two books to her credit: *Women & Development* and *Youth and Development*.

Professor Lalit M. **Nath**, MD, DrPH, calls himself an epidemiologist with an interest in research methods, HIV/AIDS and preventive cardiology. He was the head of the Centre for

Community Medicine at the All India Institute of Medical Sciences (AIIMS) for 17 years. He was the Dean of AIIMS for several years and finally retired as Director in 1996. He now works as a consultant. He was educated at the Doon School, Patna Medical College, All India Institute of Medical Sciences, and at the School of Public Health, Columbia University; but in actual fact, he says, he gained his real education working in the villages at Ballabhgarh and all over the Hindi-speaking belt. He has been actively working in the field of HIV since the late 1980s both nationally and internationally, being very active in promoting the involvement of NGOs in HIV/AIDS prevention. He was the Principal Investigator of the NGO AIDS Cell at AIIMS. He has served as a consultant to many organisations including WHO, UNICEF, UNDP, UNFPA, IDRC and the Micronutrient Initiative.

Acknowledgements

I wish to acknowledge the great help and support I have received from many people working on HIV and AIDS in India. My greatest thanks go to the chapter authors: Lalit M. Nath, Indrani Gupta, Emmanuel Eliot, S.C. Chawla, I. Koithra, Subash Hira, Swati Gupta, Tony Barnett and Shahid Ashraf, for sharing their experience and expertise with me, and for agreeing to write chapters for this book. Grants from the British Council, New Delhi and from the Overseas Development Administration (now the Department for International Development) India, were enormously helpful and are gratefully acknowledged; in particular the support of Alka Mukerjee of the British Council and Julia Cleves-Mosse of ODA. In addition I would like to thank Ms Shabbi Luthra of the American Embassy School for her help, Mr Satyamurti of Madras, and Ms Esha Beteille, formerly of Oxford University Press for their constant support, encouragement and practical assistance.

A special feature of this book is the candid reaction from a person living with HIV to the material in some of the chapters. I would like to express my sincere appreciation of the effort that a number of people took to ensure this part of the book.

Finally, I must acknowledge the patience, belief and help of my wife, Sujaya Misra, throughout the process of putting this book together.

Peter Godwin

O Arjuna, he who looks on all as on his own self, perceiving
the delight and suffering of others as his own, such a Yogi is
deemed the highest of all.
Bhagavad Gita, 6.32

But Tamas is born of ignorance and deludes all embodied
beings; it binds fast, O Bharata, through heedlessness,
indolence and sleep.
Bhagavad Gita, 14.8

Another Social Development Crisis?

PETER GODWIN

Poverty, poor health, illiteracy, malnutrition, child labour, population growth, gender bias: these are some of the development
crises India faces, and has faced for many years. Is there another
one, a new one, looming in the near future? Is the HIV epidemic
sufficiently severe to warrant special attention? Does it compare
with the long-standing crises?

This book is a collection of conceptual and analytical
frameworks, with reports of small-scale research findings, that
attempts to answer these questions. The chapters shape an outline
of the coming impact of the rapidly spreading HIV/AIDS
epidemic in India. The book aims to suggest some of the tools
that will be needed to shape policy and programmes in the coming decade to respond to the HIV/AIDS epidemic, and some of
the issues that will need to be addressed.

Adult Deaths in India

In India, about 1.2 million adults between the ages 15 and 45 die
each year.[1] Current projections of annual HIV-related deaths[2] are
between 100,000 and 500,000 annually, 10–40 per cent of all
current prime-age (15–45 years) adult deaths. But these are additional deaths to those recorded in the 1992–93 National Family
Health survey, since at that point relatively few of the HIV-in-

---

1. Based on age-specific mortality rates, as given in *The National Family
Health Survey 1992–93*, IIPS Bombay.
2. Based on Chin's EPIMODEL projections for India, as presented informally
to the GOI in 1994, and by both Nath and Gupta in the present volume (Chapters
2 & 4).

2   *The Looming Epidemic*

fected persons had started dying, given the time-lag between infection and death. These deaths are projected to rise as HIV spreads and the epidemic deepens. Indrani Gupta (see Chapter 4) suggests there may be over 300,000 in 2001. This would indicate a substantial increase in prime-age adult deaths. By contrast, the general increase in life expectancy from 50 for men and 49 for women to nearly 58 for men and 58 for women between 1971 and 1991 will cause an increase in adult ill-health (as longer-surviving adults succumb to the cardiovascular and other age-related diseases), but not in prime-age adult deaths; since these people will now die later than would previously have been expected. The effect of the HIV epidemic is thus quite different to the effect of the health transition. And as Eliot shows in Chapter 3 on mortality in Mumbai (Bombay), these untimely deaths have started to occur.

The Costs of Adult Illness and Death

The consequences of prime-age adult ill-health and death for families and households are dramatic and often devastating. They cover a wide range of areas, often in pairings of both direct costs and lost benefits, such as treatment costs and lost earnings during episodes of illness; diversion of labour and savings to care, burial and funeral expenses, and increased household expenses in extended family assistance (taking in of orphans, return of daughters, etc.); increased costs of education for extended family orphans, and the indirect costs of lost educational opportunity where children are withdrawn from school.[3] An earlier book, *The Economics of HIV and AIDS: the case of South and South East Asia*, described studies in Thailand, India, and Sri Lanka that have started to quantify these costs. Indrani Gupta, in Chapter 4 of the present volume, raises the critically important issue of the costs of adult illness related to HIV before death. The late T.N. Krishnan of the Centre for Development Studies, Thiruvanan-

---

3. The new World Bank Report, *Confronting AIDS: Public Priorities in a Global Epidemic*, OUP, 1997, gives some good examples of studies of the impact of adult deaths on education.

thapuram (Trivandrum), quoted, for example, that 40 per cent of new poverty in China is caused by ill-health, and that the situation is unlikely to be different in India. In addition are equally expensive 'social costs' where families and communities have to face unexpected deaths; in situations where rapid social change is already posing a challenge to traditional family and social structures, these costs can be enormous, affecting fertility, gender roles, household patterns, etc.

Gender Differentials

Women in particular often bear the greatest costs of adult ill-health and death, primarily because of the significant opportunity costs to them of their traditional roles as carers and nurturers of the ill or dying. Where attempts are being made to increase female enrolment rates in schools, for example, the costs of increased adult mortality are often absorbed first by withdrawing girls from school, either because their labour is needed, or because the expenses of schooling cannot be borne. In a study using the Human Development Index, researchers at Columbia and Harvard Universities found that the epidemic was affecting female educational attainment levels: 'Specifically, females are hurt more than males in the presence of AIDS, such that an increase of 100 cases per 100,000 population results in a decrease in the female–male [educational attainment] ratio of nearly one and a half points (where 100 represents equality of the sexes).'[4] Essentially this means that, in the presence of the epidemic, the tendency for girls to leave school earlier than boys is exacerbated.

Policy Implications of Changes in Prime-age Adult Mortality

There is little experience in the region, let alone in India, of dealing with the cumulative costs of a long-term, dramatic in-

---

4. David Bloom, Neil Bennett, Ajay Mahal and Waseem Noor: *The Impact of AIDS on Human Development,* UNDP, 1996 (mimeo).

crease in prime-age adult deaths. For policy-makers this increase poses a number of problems:

- The increase in deaths will not be distributed randomly across the country, but will tend to cluster in particular 'hot-spots': big cities, pilgrimage, trade and transportation centres, tribal and poor areas which supply migrant labour. These hot-spots will therefore experience very significant increases in adult mortality, far greater than the average national increases projected above.

- By virtue of the way HIV spreads (primarily through sexual intercourse), HIV-related ill-health and death will tend to cluster within households, where spouses infect each other and follow each other into early death, placing a severe cumulative strain upon affected households.

- The increase in prime-age adult ill-health and death will be significantly associated with an increase in poverty, both because of the increased susceptibility of the poor to the cause of this increased ill-health and death (HIV), and the lower ability of the poor to cope with the 'costs' of ill-health and death.

- There are few established structures to cope with relatively sudden increases in adult mortality: health services can respond to ill-health, but not to 'survivor assistance' for those left behind after death; social welfare services are often inadequate and social safety nets virtually non-existent, yet both will be required on a large scale.

- In addition, it is not possible to isolate and contain the increase in mortality and its effects: it would be inequitable to make provision for 'AIDS orphans', and not for all orphans; increases in hospital running costs because of a change in the nature of bed occupancy as HIV positive patients occupy increased numbers of places cannot be charged against specific illnesses; transfers for poor households cannot be based upon the cause of the poverty.

The combination, or cumulative effect of these problems is an *epidemic*. This is quite different to an outbreak of a disease, or even to a natural calamity. Both, while exacting a heavy toll of human suffering and death, are essentially limited in their extent and spread; in particular, both tend to be limited in duration. A large-scale, indefinite epidemic, such as that being caused by HIV extending over decades and spread all over the country, is, however, different in both direct and indirect effects, and in the kinds of long-term policy and programme responses it requires.

Responding to an Epidemic

There are few current public or private sector mechanisms in place, and a certain lack of capacity in civil society, to deal with this situation, though the National AIDS Control Programme of the Government of India has identified the strategic importance of reduction of impact; for many people, prevention is still the priority, and mitigation, or responding to impact, has not yet received full attention. This situation presents a particular challenge to national and state programmes, and to donors. Experience from Africa suggests that even when the effects of the epidemic become severely apparent, developing coordinated, effective national responses is not easy.

Up to now most HIV/AIDS programmes, whether government or NGO, have tended to regard HIV/AIDS as an isolated, separate issue, which must be dealt with externally, or in addition, to other health and social development programmes, and not as an integral part of the development challenge. It is essential to understand that there is nothing special about HIV/AIDS—it is just another disease; but there is something special about the epidemic of prime-age adult illness and death that the rapid and invisible spread of HIV is causing. Diseases can and will be dealt with by the medical profession through vaccines, medicines and medical or surgical treatment, and rehabilitation. But there are few organisations, institutions and models to handle massive epidemics, whether to prevent them, to slow down their spread, or to suppress them.

Specific Needs for Policy and Programmes

An epidemic requires specific responses in three areas: long-term protection of vulnerable populations; short-term relief and rehabilitation of those in crisis; and the strengthening of basic institutions against future shocks to come. Some of the specifics within these areas in which policy and large-scale, urgent programming are needed are:

• Poverty alleviation programmes targeted to areas specifically vulnerable to the spread of HIV—communities which are sources of migrant labour, for example, and ethnically or economically marginalised groups, as these will bear the major costs of increases in adult mortality.

• At the same time, social development programmes need to be developed for migrant labourers in cities or at mines, EPZs, development and infrastructural sites (construction of dams, railways, roads, etc), and overseas (maids, seamen, etc) which increase access to alternative forms of recreation, health advice and care, credit and small-scale banking, and financial services, for these are the individuals who will be most affected by, yet least able to cope with, premature illness and death.

• Programmes designed to facilitate entry into employment of young persons, particularly young women leaving school, as well as more general adolescence and youth programmes of education, counselling, and life-skill development are urgently needed, as they are the group most vulnerable (economically, psychologically and socially) to shocks and changes in household composition and roles therein as a result of adult illness and death.

• Social welfare and protection programmes to deal with increasing amounts of family and household dysfunction, destitution and collapse will be urgently required. Groups in need will include orphaned children, elderly 'orphans', and the destitute ill and dying of all ages.

• Health care reform programmes need to take particular note of the impact of increased morbidity, and the HIV-specific aspects of this morbidity, on health care systems.

* * *

In this book frameworks for analysis of these kinds of needs, and some basic data demonstrating their validity, are described.

Chapter 1 provides an overview of the main areas in which the impact of the epidemic will be felt, and why it is so important to address these issues. This overview makes the point that, while prime-age adult mortality is increasing (in some areas dramatically) as a result of HIV infection, few of these deaths are recorded or even recognised as HIV-related. Yet, because prime-age adult mortality rates are 'normally' low (around 0.2 per cent) relatively small increases in actual numbers of deaths produce relatively large changes in these rates.

In Chapter 2 the specifics of the epidemic in India are described, to set a context and framework for the rest of the book. The chapter outlines the situation in India, frankly acknowledging the problem of the lack of data about prevalence. But it makes the categorical point that, regardless of the exact numbers of HIV-infected people in India, the epidemic is already so widespread, and there are already so many infected cases, that a very serious problem exists. The chapter outlines an agenda for action, describing the steps necessary to prevent the spread of HIV in the country, and their effectiveness in India. It details some of the critical areas in which basic social welfare infrastructure will be threatened by the increased morbidity and mortality associated with the epidemic.

Chapter 3 demonstrates the actual impact of the epidemic on adult mortality. Projections from Africa show that levels of HIV infection among adults of around 20 per cent lead to 200–300 per cent increase in mortality. In this chapter, age-specific mortality data from the Mumbai Municipal Corporation are analysed to show an increase in adult mortality over the last eight years: 119 per cent for the 10- to 14-year-old age group and 175 per cent for boys in this age group. The possible connection with HIV is discussed.

In Chapter 4 the impact of the illness before death caused by the epidemic is assessed, based on an econometric survey of 167 people living with the virus. The sudden jump in the magnitude of the economic impact with actual illness makes clear the importance of planning for impact alleviation for the millions already infected. The policy and planning implications of this are enormous—we know that the epidemic will exacerbate poverty; yet here is an opportunity to prevent poverty.

Chapter 5 describes an attempt to use admission data from some Delhi Municipal Corporation hospitals, and the changes in patterns of mortality and morbidity which they reflect, to monitor the spread of HIV. Not only will this be a useful monitoring tool, bypassing the complexities and ethical difficulties of testing for HIV, but it will also be an important planning tool for health authorities, to help them adjust resources to respond to changing hospital needs.

Chapter 6 draws on a number of small-scale studies, and looks at what is known about the impact of the epidemic on the private sector. An analysis of needs and vulnerabilities is made and the response of industry examined.

Chapter 7 takes a preliminary look at the rural situation and stresses the concepts of susceptibility to the epidemic (the likelihood and socio-economic parameters of rapid growth of infections), and vulnerability to the longer-term social and economic impacts of the epidemic. The chapter makes some comparisons with Africa, where the impact of the epidemic on farming systems is now more clearly established, and suggests a significantly different pattern of both epidemic development and of long-term social and economic impact to that observed in Africa, based on a micro-view of a rural area in Rajasthan.

Finally, Chapter 8 addresses a particularly important area: gender differentials. Infection with HIV, and the ensuing morbidity and mortality, pose shocks and threats to households. Some of the socio-economic differentials in these shocks and threats have been identified by work in this volume and earlier work: poor households can ill afford to lose wage-earners, and have fewer household assets to draw upon; nuclear families seem to be more vulnerable than extended families; age and family size seem to affect vulnerability. In this chapter an analysis is made of gender differentials: ways in which women are more vulnerable than men; ways in which women's status, educational level and access to assets and services affect their ability to cope with these shocks; ways in which women's roles in households determine particular patterns of household response. Finally, with regard to women's health, while HIV is often described as a sexually transmitted disease, this is only true with respect to how it is transmitted. The nature of illness associated with HIV, and the kinds of responses necessary, are very different to those associated with other sexually transmitted diseases. The need to accommodate this analysis within policy and programmes for women's reproductive health is vital.

This book also introduces an unconventional element: at the end of several chapters a short discussion is recorded between the editor and a person living with HIV or AIDS (PLWHA), about the contents of the chapter. The intention is to anchor the conceptual and analytical work described in the chapter in the real experience of those directly affected by the virus.

CHAPTER ONE

The Making of an Epidemic:
An Overview of the Issues

PETER GODWIN

The HIV Epidemic and Mortality

One of the more serious discordancies in the literature on the HIV epidemic is the varying descriptions of HIV-related mortality, and the confusion regarding the nature of the epidemic that this suggests. In 1995, for example, the World Health Organisation's *World Health Report* (Table 1, p. 3) did not include the categories HIV or AIDS in its ranking of leading global causes of morbidity or mortality. Yet the 1993 *World Development Report* of the World Bank ranked HIV first and fourth respectively, as the cause of disease and death among men and women aged 15–44 in the demographically developing countries. The new 'AIDS in the World II' estimates that in 1995 alone 4.7 million new HIV infections occurred, and 1.9 million people developed AIDS. If those 1.9 million new AIDS cases all died within a year of developing the disease, AIDS would rank 8th, ahead of 'Falls, fires and drowning' and Measles, and just 100,000 short of Malaria, number seven in the WHO global assessment of mortality. Is the mortality associated with HIV on a serious scale, as an epidemiological and public health or social welfare issue; or is it a set of individual tragedies which have little overall impact on national and/or global mortality? How does it compare with other national or global causes of mortality and morbidity? And what kinds of health, social and economic impact will this global mortality have?

To start to answer these questions, three things need to be considered: the relationship between infection with HIV and illness and death; the ages at which illness and death occur; and the nature of health and medical reporting and epidemiology systems.

To deal with the first point; the relationship between infection with HIV and illness and death. The *World Health Report 1995* notes that '... there will be a huge increase in the number of AIDS cases. It is estimated that 4 million adults and children have developed AIDS since the start of the pandemic. The cumulative total [of "AIDS cases"] is projected to reach nearly 10 million by the year 2000.' But what is an 'AIDS case'? In Europe and America most people with HIV progress eventually to a clinical state recognised and diagnosed as being AIDS. In many parts of the developing world, however, this progress never takes place, as people infected with HIV tend to die before they develop AIDS.[1] Similarly, what is an 'AIDS death'? It could be a specific death from clinically manifest AIDS, but it could also, and it is often used thus, be a statistical, or notional death estimated or projected to occur as a result of HIV infection: a death not necessarily directly attributable to clinical AIDS, but rather to a more common cause, resulting however from infection with HIV, and thus a compromised immune system. This is further complicated by the fact that there are no 'HIV deaths': infection with HIV does not, in and of itself, cause death.

It is thus important to distinguish between morbidity and mortality arising as a result of infection with HIV—whether diagnosed or estimated and projected—and morbidity and mortality directly arising from the presence of clinical AIDS.[2] In the first case, the WHO Report is correct: the number of recorded 'AIDS deaths' is still relatively low; the numbers arising from the second

---

1. Charles F. Gilks: 'The clinical challenge of the HIV epidemic in the developing world', *The Lancet*, Vol 342, Oct 1993.

2. A third term, 'HIV disease' to cover both situations has been coined, but is not widely used yet. cf Gilks op. cit.

case, however, are a matter of very grave concern. They signify perhaps the largest change in young adult mortality in the last 50 years, and a change in the wrong direction.

The second cause of confusion is the age-specificity of illness and death. Most illness and death is clustered at the beginning of life, in babies and children, and at the end of life, among the old, as part of, or leading to, 'natural' death. The top four causes of death in the WHO top ten list, accounting for 56 per cent of all deaths in the list, are heart disease (affecting mainly the elderly), respiratory infections under 5 years of age, cerebrovascular diseases (again, primarily of the elderly) and diarrhoea under age 5. Most HIV-related illness and death, largely because of how HIV is transmitted—through sex, occurs among young adults; 60 per cent of global infections among women are estimated to occur by age 20.

To understand the impact of HIV on mortality, therefore, it is important secondly, to distinguish between illness and death among children and the aged, where morbidity and mortality rates are already high, and illness and death among prime-age adults, where morbidity and mortality rates are usually low. In India, for example, the crude death rate among children under 5 is 23.3 per 1000 population; for people 60–64 it is 22.8; for those above 70 it is 95; while for people 20–24 it is 2.6—almost one-tenth of under 5 mortality, and only one-thirty-seventh of over 70 mortality. This means that changes in mortality rates have very different effects, depending on the ages at which they occur, as much of the rest of this book describes. A relatively small change in the number of actual deaths compared to the total population, if clustered in the young adult age group, could significantly change the death rate in that age group. Yet it is this group in which the greatest reductions in mortality have taken place in the last few decades: increases in life-expectancy have meant that in India the probability of dying between 15 and 30 years of age was reduced by almost 50 per cent between 1941 and 1970, for both males and females. As we shall see later, changes in the death rate in that age group have important social and economic consequences. Talking of illness, let alone early death, the World Bank says: 'The consequences of adult ill-health extend far beyond increased consumption of medical care and range from dramatic effects on the health of other household members to subtle but probably costly effects on the efficiency with which a society organises its currently healthy workers.... By robbing the individual and therefore the household, the community, and the employer of time and resources, adult ill-health limits the development potential of the societies which it burdens.'[3]

Finally, for many reasons, illness, and particularly deaths, directly resulting from infection with HIV are not recognised, let alone reported, as having any connection with HIV. As noted above, the actual cause of death (or of illness) in many developing countries is often an identifiable communicable disease: pneumonia or tuberculosis, for example. Such a situation, even if the sero-status of the individual is known, is usually recorded as resulting from the communicable disease. The recognised evidence of this is the recorded increase in TB around the world; while much of this is due to the emergence of drug-resistant strains of TB, WHO estimates that in Africa at least 25 per cent of this increase is HIV attributable.[4] In Chiang Rai, in Northern Thailand, a recent study found that: 'Following a steady decline in reported TB from 1982 through 1991, the incidence of TB increased sharply. TB ... data from Chiang Rai Hospital ... indicated a steady and rapid increase in the number and proportion of HIV-seropositive TB patients from four (1.5 per cent of all TB patients) in 1990 to 207 (45.5 per cent) in 1994.'[5] In many countries where the presence of HIV is not widely recognised or admitted, there may well appear to be no particular reason to

3. Feachem et al.: *The Health of Adults in the Developing World*, Oxford University Press, New York, 1992.

4. Dermot Maher (WHO) in an ODA funded special supplement on TB in Africa, *Africa Health*, 19 (1), 17–24, 1996.

5. Hideki Yanai et al.: 'Rapid increase in HIV-related tuberculosis, Chiang Rai, Thailand, 1990–1994', *AIDS* 10: 527–31, 1996.

check sero-status, which makes the recording of any connection with HIV even more unlikely (even where there is no other known cause, and the actual cause of death remains unknown). If we add to this the tendency of both the infected and the health worker to keep HIV infection or AIDS secret or confidential, to avoid discrimination and stigmatisation, it is understandable why such reporting of illness and death potentially related to HIV pervades national systems, reducing significantly the reported occurrence of HIV or AIDS. Finally, the length of time between infection with HIV and serious illness and death (several years at the least), and the lack of any visible indicators of HIV status, tend to discourage obvious connections between HIV status and illness and death. In many people's eyes, HIV is much more likely to be associated with lifestyle than with symptoms.

The Impact of Adult Mortality

What then is clear about HIV-related morbidity and mortality? Little is known so far about Asia; and even less about India. Recent work from Africa, however, estimates that by the end of the century 'AIDS will double the number of deaths and the crude death rate in many of the countries most affected by the epidemic, as compared with the levels expected in the absence of AIDS'.[6] This work goes on to estimate 'a 20 per cent seroprevalence is likely to cause a 3- to 5-fold increase in prime-age adult mortality ... among groups where the seroprevalence rises to between 45 and 90 per cent, mortality might rise by a factor of 10.' It concludes: 'Infant /child mortality and life expectancy, which had experienced a 30- to 40-year period of improvement in many of these countries, are already showing the impact of AIDS and will suffer further setbacks in coming years.

---

6. Barney Cohen & James Trussel, eds: *Preventing and Mitigating AIDS in Sub-Saharan Africa: Research and Data Priorities for the Social and Behavioural Sciences*, National Academy Press, Washington DC, p. 218, 1996.

Development programs and child survival projects, which have used such measures as indicators of program impact, will be forced to attempt to factor out the effect of AIDS or develop alternative indicators.'

In Asia, detailed work projecting the effects of the epidemic has only really been done in Thailand; though a number of basic projections exist for India, Hong Kong, Cambodia, and some other countries.

In Thailand,[7] projections suggest that if the epidemic progresses unchecked, by the year 2005 annual HIV-related deaths will be 83,000; and even if ambitious prevention programme targets are reached (such as an increase in condom use rates from the current 30 per cent to 90 per cent, and the reduction of STD rates from 4.5/1000 to 1.3/1000), annual deaths related to HIV will still be 57,000. A recent study in Chiang Mai Province found that age-specific mortality rates had dramatically increased among young adult men and women; by nearly 600 per cent among men, putting them significantly higher than child mortality rates.[8] Detailed projections for the impact of AIDS on children have also been prepared in Thailand.[9] These estimate, that by the year 2005, 7500 children a year will be dying as a result of HIV infection against an estimated 730 in 1990, and 3800 in 1994. 'By the end of the decade, however, a child death resulting from AIDS will no longer be a rare event, and will in fact be the major contributing cause of child deaths, comprising 33 per cent of all deaths that occur under the age of 5 years, and 25 per cent of deaths in the first year of life .... The effects on mortality rates will be significant. In the absence of AIDS, infant mortality is projected to decline by almost 30 per cent over the decade. However, if the AIDS epidemic proceeds as projected ... [F]or infant

---

7. National Economic and Social Development Board Working group, Bangkok.

8. Peter Godwin, Emmanuel Eliot, S.C. Chawla & Im-em, forthcoming.

9. Tim Brown & Werasit Sittitrai: *The Impact of HIV on Children in Thailand*, Thai Red Cross Society, 1995.

mortality, rates in 2000 will be at 1991 levels, while under-5 mortality rates in the year 2000 will be higher than 1990 levels.'[10]

In India very few estimates of the prevalence of infection with HIV and the impact on mortality have been made. One set of projections, prepared with EPIMODEL[11] in 1994, however, do suggest some orders of magnitude for national HIV-related mortality. On a low scenario, starting with a figure of 500,000 cumulative HIV infections in 1992, annual 'AIDS cases' are calculated at 25,000 in 1994, rising to 110,000 by the year 2000. This would be about 10 per cent of current annual prime-age adult mortality. On a moderate scenario, estimating three-quarters of a million HIV infections in 1992, annual 'AIDS cases' would be 190,000 by 2000. The high scenario, estimating HIV infections to be 1 million in 1992, gives 100,000 cumulative 'AIDS cases' by 1994, and 300,000 annual 'AIDS cases' by 2000—nearly 30 per cent of current prime-age adult mortality.

Reference has already been made to age-specific mortality rates in India. As Eliot shows in Chapter 3, mortality rates are changing in areas where HIV has spread. While the direct connection between these changes and HIV is very difficult to prove, the correlations with causes of deaths, and the age groups in which the changes are largely taking place, are highly suggestive.

Interpretation of these meagre data suggests four conclusions:

- The spread of HIV in India will produce an increase in mortality among prime-age adults (15–45).
- Prime-age adult mortality is generally low; therefore this increase will be significant, even at low levels.
- The elements of this mortality (proximate causes) are many; consequently the contribution of HIV to the increase in mortality is often overlooked.

---

10. Boonchalaksi Wathinee and Guest Philip: '*AIDS and children: Prospects for the year 2000*, IPSR Publication No. 168, Institute for Population and Social Research, Mahidol University, Thailand, July 1993.

11. An informal presentation to GOI by James Chin.

- The delay between infection with HIV and mortality is long; a
  further reason for overlooking the connection with HIV.

These conclusions are important, since they form the basis for
serious strategising and programming. This book aims to
elucidate the elements of this change in adult mortality, and the
likely impact it will have in India.

The Immediate Impact: The Supply of and Demand for Health Care

Dr Lalit Nath, former Director, All India Institute of Medical
Sciences (AIIMS), New Delhi, has identified eight areas in which
the HIV/AIDS epidemic will impact on the health system:[12]
managing waste disposal in hospitals; the adoption of universal
precautions in hospitals; managing blood in and outside hospitals;
training of health care providers (diagnosis, management, attitudes, etc, and diagnosis not only for AIDS, but also for increase
in HIV-related common illness); the availability of drugs,
medicines and supplies; provision of counselling services; pro-
viding terminal care; and overloading of communicable disease
care at primary care level. This list combines both largely
HIV/AIDS-specific impacts (such as the blood supply and
universal precautions), and impacts arising from an increase in
adult morbidity whatever the cause (such as availability of
drugs). Yet little is known, either in India or anywhere else in the
world, about the scope and scale of these impacts. Some preliminary studies in Africa, the Pacific and Sri Lanka into some of
these areas suggest that the impact will be very significant indeed, particularly at a time when many health care systems are
undergoing reform, to make them more financially viable and
sustainable.

---

12. See Chapter 2 in this volume.

Studies in Sri Lanka, for example, examined the cost-benefits of introducing universal precautions, disposable needles and syringes, pooling of blood for screening etc, both for current HIV prevalence levels and for projected levels, and suggested guidelines for policy in these matters.[13] Data from the Christian Medical College, Vellore, have been used to estimate the increased cost arising from increased use and disposal of materials etc., of surgical procedures on patients known to be HIV positive.[14] In the Pacific, estimates suggest that the health care costs for a person living with HIV or AIDS are more than ten times the present average per capita expenditure on health care and several times the per capita income.[15] Similar studies from Thailand, Indonesia and India have made the same point.[16] Any chronic illness in an adult, however, will produce the same effect; considering that most adults make little charge against the health system annually as long as they remain healthy. The significance of these studies is in the fact that they relate to an increase in young adult illness and death; the costs therefore imply an expected net increase in national expenditure on health care.

Two other changes in national health systems in Asia compound the effects that increased morbidity from HIV and AIDS will produce, yet also provide a context within which the issue can be approached. The first is the movement towards 'the health transition',[17] and the second the movement towards health care reform. The health transition refers to the shift towards a greater prominence of diseases suffered by adults and the elderly: some of these are growing in prevalence as a result of demographic changes (increased numbers of adults surviving longer), others

13. Bloom & Godwin: *The Economics of AIDS: the Case of South and South-East Asia*, OUP 1997.

14. Dr T. Jacob John, personal communication.

15. Ahlburg et al.: 'Health care costs and HIV/AIDS in the Pacific', *Pacific Health Dialog* 2: 2, 1995.

16. Bloom & Lyons: *The Economic Implications of AIDS*, UNDP New Delhi, 1993.

17. Feachem et al.: op. cit.

are becoming more widespread as a result of changing lifestyles; both are more costly and resource-intensive to deal with. The general increase in life expectancy in India from 50 for men and 49 for women to nearly 58 for men and 58 for women between 1971 and 1991 will cause an increase in adult ill-health (as longer-surviving adults succumb to cardiovascular and other age-related diseases), but not in prime-age (15–45 years) adult deaths, since these people will now die later than would earlier have been expected. The effect of the HIV epidemic is thus quite different to the effect of the health transition (see Eliot in Chapter 3 of this volume).

Similarly, the trend towards reform of health systems, and particularly the financing of health care, is a response to the growing costs of health care, and the increasing demand for health services that development has brought. 'Many countries have not been able to sustain their prior commitments to either the provision or the financing of health care.'[18] Prioritising health care expenditure is difficult, as differing conceptions of needs influence policy. In India, between 1974/75 and 1990/91 a number of changes in the prioritising of health care took place, reflecting changing policies. While per capita government spending on medical and public health components increased in real terms by 43 per cent, expenditure on family planning increased by 150 per cent, on water supply and sanitation by 166 per cent and on child and handicapped welfare by 596 per cent.[19] Overall the share of medical and public health 'slipped' from 62 per cent of government expenditure to 49 per cent in this period. Of course, much of this change was counterbalanced by massive increases in private sector health spending.[20] These figures, however, demonstrate the necessity of adequate policy and planning. It is

18. David Dunlop & Jo Martins eds: *An International Assessment of Health Care Financing*, World Bank, 1995.

19. K.N. Reddy & V. Selvaraju: *Health Care Expenditure by Government in India*, Seven Hills Publications, 1994.

20. Peter Berman & M.E. Khan eds., *Paying for India's Health Care*, Sage Publications, New Delhi, 1993.

critical that the effects of increased morbidity and mortality, occurring in very specific age and population groups, and with
specific geographical intensity, resulting from the spread of HIV,
are factored adequately into national policies for health services
as they evolve under these two imperatives: the health transition
and the financing of health care.

Productivity: Is It at Risk?

A healthy and educated labour force is critical to sustained
economic development, both at the macro-economic level, and at
the micro-level, with respect to individual businesses. 'Private
domestic investment, combined with rapidly growing human
capital, were the principal engines of growth' says the World
Bank, explaining East Asia's economic success.[21] What impact,
then, will a change in morbidity and mortality amongst a labour
force have? As has been shown in the Introduction, there will be
substantial changes in mortality and morbidity produced by the
HIV epidemic, and these changes will be particularly clustered
among young adults, who make up the bulk of the labour force in
India as elsewhere. Evidence from earlier work by Bloom and
Godwin (op. cit.) show that these changes do not appear to have
a macro-economic effect; are they likely to have a micro-
economic impact, on individual businesses? A study in Madras
found that a single case of AIDS in one company accounted for 3
per cent of total work hours lost over three years by that company
and two others; this compared to 11 per cent lost due to TB
(number of cases not known, but surely more than 1), 62 per cent
due to viral fever, and 8 per cent due to accidents and injuries.[22]
Chapter 6 in this volume describes some other work along these
lines.

●

21. *The East Asian Miracle: Economic Growth and Public Policy*, a World
Bank Policy Research Report, 1993.
22. ILO Study with EFSI, L. Tegmo-Reddy, personal communication.

Two factors can be identified as important in this analysis: the level of risk a business faces, and what mechanisms it has for responding to this risk. The level of risk is mainly determined by the vulnerability of the labour force to infection with HIV, the prevalence of HIV in the environment in which the labour force lives, works and plays, and the distribution of possible infection within the labour force. The response mechanisms vary from neglect to various forms of health benefit schemes. Both are vulnerable to increases in health care costs; even neglect, in that the pain of neglect is felt more widely in the community, and burdens other public sector mechanisms.

Gender: Is There a Special Case for Women?

Chapter 8 in this volume considers, in some detail, gender differentials in Indian society and the special case for women arising from these. Here, three points will be emphasised. Firstly, the ability to protect oneself from HIV infection, and to cope with the consequences if one is unable to protect oneself, involve major choices and decisions about lifestyle and personal behaviour. Wherever people are disempowered, through lack of education, lack of personal or social control of their behaviour, poverty, or access to support and services, their ability to make these choices and decisions will be limited. In India today, many people of both sexes are disempowered in exactly these ways—but women, in general, more so. The facts, detailed in Chapter 8, make plain that women go to school less, are employed less, earn less, are more circumscribed in their behaviour by social taboos, and have less access to services, than men.

Secondly, as is dealt with in more detail by Tony Barnett in Chapter 7 of this volume, the particular nature of migration and mobility in India probably puts women at special risk. Decosis suggests that it is not the origin or the destination of migration, but the social disruption which characterises certain types of migration which determines vulnerability to HIV.[23] Very little is known about these aspects of migration in India—an area which requires urgent research and analysis. But it is not unlikely that the female companions of male migrants subject to this kind of 'social disruption', wherever they may be living—in the village from which the migrant sets out, in the urban slum where he temporarily lives, or in a semi-urban new settlement—will suffer very severely from the epidemic.

Finally, the lack of support and welfare services for women, whether in cases of ill-health, poverty, or social and psychological need, urgently needs to be addressed. As studies of prostitution have shown, women in need face stark choices. As the epidemic spreads, the numbers of women in need will grow considerably.

The Impact on the Future: Children, and the Education System

A path-breaking piece of work in Thailand has assessed the impact of the epidemic on Thailand's children.[24] The study found that in 1994 approximately 5,900 children were orphaned (defined as losing their mothers) by AIDS. By the year 2000, this number will have grown to 23,000 a year. By this time nearly half a million (450,000) living children will have mothers who are either HIV-infected, or have died of AIDS; perhaps twice that number will have lost their father. Very little is known about the likely impact on children in India, where, since much larger numbers of people are infected than in Thailand, much larger numbers of children will be affected; though, as mentioned earlier, the new World Bank Report, 'Confronting AIDS: Public Priorities in a Global Epidemic', (OUP, 1997) describes the effects of young

---

23. J. Decosis et al.: 'Migration and AIDS', *The Lancet*, Sept 23, 1995.
24. Tim Brown and Werasit Sittitrai: *The Impact of HIV on Children in Thailand*, Thai Red Cross Society, 1995.

adult deaths and orphaning on child nutrition and education in some detail.

Shaffer, drawing on the experience of very severely affected parts of East Africa, has identified three ways in which the epidemic will have its impact upon the education system: on the supply of education, the demand for education, and the quality of education.[25] Supply is affected as teachers become infected, ill and eventually die; demand is affected as schoolchildren become ill and die, or, more immediately, are withdrawn from school because of increased illness and death in their families; and quality changes as schools are forced to play a stronger 'counselling' role, responding to the needs of large numbers of distressed and psychologically traumatised children who have experienced the collapse of their families and communities. Little is known about whether parts of India will experience the levels of seroprevalence in which the education system is as seriously affected as Shaffer describes. One scenario, however, certainly suggests that this could happen—if the infection spreads through labour or seasonal migration from high prevalence areas such as the great cities into poor rural communities, where schools are few and often small, and teachers fewer. If one teacher dies in a community that has only two or three, this is as serious a blow to that community's education system as if hundreds died in Delhi.

More immediately, there are two specific questions which the education sector in India would do well to consider:

• Are children in schools being taught what they need to know to deal with a huge new epidemic in their country, and in their cities? This does not mean merely 'sex education', or instruction on how to use a condom; but rather helping them to develop the values and understanding which will prepare them to face illness and death, fear, discrimination and stigmatisation, loneliness and despair—not only for themselves, if they

---

25. See Sheldon Shaffer in Tim Brown and Werasit Sittitrai, *The Impact of HIV on Children in Thailand,* op. cit.

are unfortunate enough to become infected, but also for their family or friends, and for others who become infected.

• Are headmistresses and headmasters equipped to deal with a situation which they will certainly have to face (if they haven't already had to do so)—where one of their students, or one of the teachers, becomes HIV positive?

Conclusion: Is There a Time Frame?

The combination of a significant increase in age-specific morbidity and mortality occurring over a significant period of time into the future; the psychological, medical, social, organisational and economic 'costs' resulting from this increase; and the effects on populations and sub-populations upon whom these costs are likely to most severely fall, is creating a serious epidemic for India. As this overview has shown, this epidemic will occur mainly among young adults, will seriously overstretch health care and social welfare systems, and will be most devastating for the poor, and for women. Furthermore, this epidemic will last into the next two decades at least.

Little is known about the likely time scale of the epidemic. The new edition of *AIDS in the World* offers a long-term scenario even more frightening than that of current conventional thinking, projecting the wide spread of the virus into very large numbers of the 'low-vulnerability' general population in all countries; perhaps taking decades to do this; '... the global experience of HIV/AIDS is likely only beginning. Available data suggest the possibility that a decrease in annual incidence of new HIV infections may occur; the warning must be sounded that this may only be the "lull before the storm" and that this apparently hopeful outcome may only presage the next phase in a long, sustained struggle with the pandemic.'[26]

---

26. Jonathan Mann and Daniel Tarantola eds: *AIDS in the World II*, OUP, 1996.

There is some likelihood of a vaccine, or an effective and affordable cure being developed in the next decade or two. But even if a vaccine or cure is discovered, there is little expectation that sufficient changes will have taken place in health systems in the developing world to make effective coverage of all in need a real possibility within the same time scale. Measles vaccine has been available for thirty years, yet measles is still one of the biggest killers of children in India.[27]

But a more important consideration is the consequences of waiting for a vaccine or cure. Although prevention programmes have been shown to be effective to some extent, with specific population groups and under specific circumstances, the practical experience of the last ten years suggests convincingly that, with what we know of the speed with which the virus can spread, there is little real likelihood that prevention can be extended on a scale necessary to seriously interrupt or interdict this spread of the virus in many countries in Asia—India among them—until infection rates reach similar levels to those in parts of Africa. This is especially the case in view of the great constraints under which health programmes function in many countries.

Even if prevention programmes were to be launched immediately on the necessary scale, or, even more fantastically, the virus were suddenly to disappear, in many countries—India among them—there are already a sufficient number of people infected, many of them likely never to be identified, so that the impact of the epidemic will continue for several years to come. In Thailand, for example, projections have been made for the next decade: even if the targets for the ambitious prevention programme are met 100 per cent by the year 2005, 500,000 infections will have been averted, but 450,000 new infections will still have occurred, doubling the current number of infections; in addition, annual HIV-related deaths will still be 57,000. In many parts of India, which is estimated to have more than four times as many infections as Thailand, the number of infections will continue to grow

27. *World Health Report, 1996,* WHO SEARO.

for many years. Even were it not to, as the Thailand example shows, the impact of the epidemic will continue to grow, and there is nothing we can do to stop it.

There is, in this respect, a striking similarity with the development experience of population growth, and what is called the population momentum, where because of the large numbers of children already born, populations continue to grow significantly for a while, even if birth rates fall sharply. This apparent paradox, whether in population or in the HIV epidemic, is essentially a result of lack of anticipation; and anticipation is not expensive. This is the reality which the epidemic has presented to us.

* * *

Discussion: The Personal Face of the Epidemic

PG: Satya, you have seen more and more friends, colleagues and contemporaries die as a result of HIV over the last two years. But have other community, family or society members noticed the increase in young people dying yet, do you think?

S: Most direct family members *do* notice that the deaths of individuals are due to the complications of HIV. Yet these family members, like People Living with HIV or AIDS (PLWHA), have had to remain anonymous, silent, fearing social reactions, fearing that the deceased's property may not be returned (there are incidents like this in Madras), and, worst of all, that the funeral may not be carried out if the death certificate states 'Died due to AIDS'. In fact, whenever a person has died of AIDS, the family members request the physician not to mention this in the death certificate. The necessity to remain anonymous is an indication of the very real oppression which the infected and affected people face—from other people. Peter, it's a vicious circle—until people can be easier about their family or community members who have died of AIDS, we will remain hidden and be 'others'.

PG: So you're saying that the denial of the implications and reality of HIV and AIDS at the personal level carries over to community and national level. No one wants to know about or accept this?

S: Yes. The deaths of young adults are not recognised or admitted as AIDS-related. Since PLWHA die mainly of TB, or diarrhoeal disease, it goes in the record as TB, or diarrhoea. Also, because of the long incubation of HIV disease, it makes it even more difficult for people to recognise that these deaths are due to HIV or AIDS.

PG: We all spend a lot of time talking about 'socio-economic impact'. In your experience, what effects do these deaths have?

S: In my personal experience, I would classify the impact as follows:

- Income: the loss of a PLWHA in his/her prime leads to increased poverty in the family. Since laws and customs restrict women's income-generating capacity, poverty in the family is exacerbated with the death of a male head. Women are unable to compensate for lost income by taking on the same or similar earning strategies.

- The funeral of the deceased family member: after exhausting all their resources before death, the people left behind have to really struggle for funeral expenses: anything from Rs 3,000 to 10,000. It is very difficult for people to borrow money for this, as most of them (the ones I've seen and spoken to) have already borrowed money from as many people as they can, and sold all their property, for treatment before death.

- Household management: things like paying rent, electricity bills, and other essential expenses.

- Food supply: the food supply, and so the nutrition of the family goes down. This is a very serious issue, for in most of the cases that I've seen the survivors are themselves positive. These PLWHA can no longer afford the proper quality of food, which means their health starts to deteriorate faster.

- Finally, the effect of the death of an adult on the children: this has not been very widely noticed as far as I know, but it is starting to happen. There are a few instances which I have come across where the child or children have been removed from school, either to take care of someone at home, or to be sent into employment to support the family.

Please remember, this analysis should not be considered complete. It is purely my own personal experience and observation of people with HIV/AIDS over the past few years.

CHAPTER TWO

The Epidemic in India: An Overview

LALIT M. NATH

Introduction

The Nation's Response

HIV infection is now common in India; exactly what the prevalence is, is not really known, but it can be stated without any fear of being wrong that the infection is widespread and has been reported from almost every part of the country. There is also ample evidence that the virus is no longer confined to segments that were considered at special risk. From being found in commercial sex workers and injecting-drug users, it is spreading rapidly into those segments that society in India does not recognise as being at risk. Housewives and white collar workers are now being diagnosed as HIV positive or even as suffering from AIDS. AIDS is beginning to come out of the closet.[1]

Responses to the epidemic can still be thought of in three fairly well-defined groups. The first category comprises those few scientists and occasional NGOs who have been trying hard to convince decision-makers and the public that there is an urgent need to take action to control the HIV/AIDS pandemic.[2] The National AIDS Control Organisation (NACO) with its committed leaders also falls into this category. The message from this group does not seem to be taken too seriously either by health decision-makers, politicians or even by the public. This has prevented a

1. 'AIDS striking home', *India Today*, 15 March, 1997.
2. *Talking AIDS, Stopping AIDS*, Film produced by IAPSM and the NGO AIDS Cell, AIIMS.

more serious appraisal of the facts as propagated by the serious scientists worried about the possible impact of the epidemic.

The next category are the health decision-makers in general. They are characterised by persons who either do not really believe the horrendous picture being painted by the first group or who genuinely believe that Indians are different and 'it can't happen here'! One feels that there are many decision-makers who think the problem will go away if they close their eyes, or that they have many other priorities and this problem will have to wait until the other priorities have been attended to; or even those who think that all that is needed has been done now that the people have been told to use condoms to protect themselves!

The third group comprises the general public. Most of them have never really thought about the problem and are too busy existing from day to day to worry about abstract issues; and AIDS is certainly an abstract issue in India. With no societal knowledge of the disease, no cultural or traditional beliefs about AIDS, it remains as yet as distant as the men walking on the moon. The few who have the inclination or the leisure to think, probably feel that HIV/AIDS is certainly a problem but it cannot happen to 'nice' people and so it is a problem only of 'those' people—'those' being defined in terms of individual bias and prejudice.

Given this scenario it is obvious that the nation's response is still sub-optimal. The health decision-makers' actions seem to be knee jerk reflexes driven by donor prodding, and the people's response seems to be apathy and business as usual.

The Situation in India: The Likely Picture

Estimates about HIV Prevalence

Several estimates have been made about the prevalence of HIV infection in the country. WHO's previous Global Programme on AIDS (GPA) and now UNAIDS have been predicting that India will soon have the dubious distinction of being the epicentre of the HIV/AIDS pandemic in the world.[3] Another frequently quoted estimate was published by a group of authors from the GPA and the National AIDS Control Organisation (NACO).[4] According to this paper India had approximately 1,750,000 adult HIV positive persons. At the end of 1995 NACO suggested a seroprevalence of 1.7 per 1000 for the country; this works out to an estimated 1.5 million persons who were HIV positive as of the end of 1995.[5]

The South East Asia Regional Office of the World Health Organisation (SEARO/WHO) has estimated in March 1997 that there are 2.5 million HIV positive persons in India.[6] Calculations made by Professor T. Jacob John of Vellore estimated that there were 4.48 million infected persons in the country.[7] NACO as of the end of March 1998 has reported 74,960 HIV positive cases out of the 3.29 million samples screened.[8]

It is unfortunate that we do not have a well-accepted and dependable estimate of the HIV prevalence in the country. The estimates that have been made are inevitably best guesses. While sporadic information is available about some special 'at risk' groups, mostly urban, we really do not have a good estimate of rural prevalence. As over 70 per cent of the population of India lives in the rural areas, the lack of estimates of rural prevalence seriously compromises the validity of most of the common estimates of the HIV load in the country.

3.   Peter Piot: UNAIDS, MAP, Vancouver.

4.   Burton A, Thierry E.M. in Shiv Lal: 'Estimation of Adult HIV Prevalence as of the end of 1994 in India', *Ind. J. Pub. Health*, 39: 79–85, 1995.

5.   *National AIDS Control Programme India, Country Scenario Update*, NACO, MOHFW, Dec. 1995.

6.   WHO, SEARO: *AIDS update March 7, 1997.*

7.   T. Jacob John: 'Estimating the burden of HIV infection in India', *Round table on HIV/AIDS Surveillance in India*, Network for Child Development and Association for Health, Environment and Development, New Delhi, 1996.

8.   NACO: 'Surveillance for HIV infection/AIDS Cases in India', *Report up to 31 March 1998.*

The estimates range from about 1.5 million HIV positive individuals in India currently, to as many as almost 4.5 million. It is likely that the true value lies somewhere within this range. The exact figure remains an academic issue and has little programmatic implication. It is a very large number, even by Indian standards. But not knowing the exact number of HIV positive persons in the country must not be allowed to be an excuse for delaying vigorous public health action. The interventions required to be put in place will not change whether the actual number turns out to be one million or even five million; once we are dealing with such very large numbers, we have a very serious problem. No matter where exactly the true figure lies, there is no contesting the fact that there are a lot of HIV positive persons in India and that it is essential that health decision-makers take immediate steps to minimise the spread of HIV today and cope with the expected onrush of new AIDS patients.

It must be kept in mind that with a total population close to the billion mark, even a small prevalence can add up to a large number of people. Though there are a lot of HIV positive persons in India, overall the prevalence is still low and much lower than in many other nations. India is still in the second phase of the epidemic.[9] This does not mean we can afford to be complacent, it only implies that preventive measures are likely to be very cost effective.

At the current stage of our knowledge we can assume that almost all HIV positive persons will eventually develop AIDS and then succumb to some infection. Any death, especially of someone in the beginning of his productive and family life is deplorable. The cost of loss of economic activity and wasted expenditure on training and nurturing the person concerned can be measured by economists, but the cost in terms of pain and suffering for the family and the community is difficult to quantify but is nevertheless very significant. What is even more important from the point of view of the impact upon the health system and

---

9. UNDP, as quoted in 'Time to Act', United Nations, Fiji, p. 21, 1996.

the economy, is that many more people will have repeated episodes of illness, many of which will require hospitalisation. It is this cost of medical care coupled with a concomitant loss of income that drives most families with a patient of HIV/AIDS to penury.

Reporting and Estimating HIV/AIDS Deaths and Their Impact

The epidemic in India was first detected ten years ago[10] and deaths in substantial numbers are now being reported. Up to the end of March 1998, 5,204 cases of AIDS have been reported to the authorities. Of course, this is a gross underestimate of actual AIDS cases or even deaths. Salunke, using EPIMODEL, has suggested that by the end of 1996 in Maharashtra alone, there have been 341,623 deaths from AIDS.[11]

For a variety of reasons all deaths due to AIDS are not reported; AIDS is not a notifiable disease under the law; many doctors do not report the diagnosis of AIDS to protect the patient's family; finally as some Mumbai-based doctors held during a meeting in Pune, 'why should they bother to report a case of AIDS when it had become such a usual and almost commonplace experience!'[12]

It is also true that most cases of AIDS are not diagnosed. Testing facilities are not available at all places. The clinical criteria for diagnosing AIDS are not well known in India. And finally the index of suspicion is still low. Infectious diseases are common and finding a lung or meningeal infection or a flourishing thrush does not automatically trigger alarm bells. Many, if not most deaths, including AIDS deaths, occur at home, and if this is outside an urban area, registration of deaths are irregular at best. The terminal event may not be attended by a qualified doctor.

---

10. T. Jacob John, op. cit.

11. Salunke S.R.: Presentation during Expert Group on HIV Estimates, 1997.

12. International Symposium on 'Biomedical, clinical and social research issues in HIV infection and their policy implications', 2–4 May, National AIDS Research Institute, Pune, India, 1994.

The Ministry of Health and Family Welfare reported that only 14.28 per cent of all deaths in the country were medically certified.[13] For all these reasons the reported cases are just a very small proportion of the total mortality from this disease.

Cohort studies have shown that the mean time from infection to developing AIDS is 9.8 years.[14] A recent report suggests that this may even be true for perinatal HIV/AIDS.[15] There have also been suggestions that in the developing world the disease progresses more rapidly[16] and many of us believe that in countries where the health care facilities are severely limited the mean survival time after developing clinical AIDS is shorter than in areas where more acute infection control and terminal care facilities are common. But just as estimates of prevalence are uncertain, reliable estimates of the annual expected mortality from AIDS for India over the next few years are not available. It is thus difficult to accurately predict the exact patient care load that will evolve over the next few years due to the HIV epidemic.

The World Bank, for instance, estimated that its support for the interventions programmed through NACO had the potential for averting 300,000 deaths.[17] All these persons would have needed hospital care for HIV-related illness especially during the last year or two of life, and therefore a rough estimate of the load on the medical system can be calculated. If a patient of HIV infection leading to AIDS needs six admissions for HIV-related

---

13. *Health Information of India*, Central Bureau of Health Intelligence, DGHS, MOHFW, p. 189, 1994.

14. P. Bacheti & A.R. Moss: 'Incubation period of AIDS in San Francisco', *Nature*, 338: 251–3, 1989.

15. H.X. Barnhart, M.B. Caldwell, P. Thomas, et al. and the Paediatric Spectrum of Disease Clinical Consortium: 'Naturally History of Human Immunodeficiency Virus Disease in Peri-natally Infected Children: an analysis from the Paediatric Spectrum of Disease Project'. *Paediatrics*, 97: 710–16 as quoted in Evidence-Based Medicine, January/February p. 26, 1997.

16. John Stover: 'The impact of HIV/AIDS on adult and child mortality in the developing world', *Health Transition Review*, supplement to vol. 4, 1004, p. 49, 1994.

17. World Bank, New Delhi

illness during his/her lifetime before finally succumbing, and each admission is of about two weeks with a longer terminal admission, then each person with AIDS would need about 100 hospital bed days. This would come to a staggering increased demand of 30 million bed days, which the NACO programme hopes to avert.

As no programme can be expected to be totally effective, if 300,000 deaths are prevented, the actual deaths that might have occurred can be expected to be much greater. According to NACO, India had by the end of 1995, 590,000 hospital beds which works out to 215 million bed days annually. HIV/AIDS would by these calculations be expected to tie up between 15 and 30 per cent of these. As is the case in Africa,[18] one major effect of the epidemic may be to displace other types of patients from needed hospital care.

Some Projections

In a paper on the possible economic consequences of the HIV epidemic on India,[19] the assumption was made that mortality would be distributed as 20, 30, 30 and 20 per cent in the four successive quartiles. This is an estimate based on our under-standing of the epidemiology of the disease, taking into consideration that the mean survival interval is about ten years. (Of course if the pattern of deaths followed a normal distribution the figures would perhaps be a little greater in the second and third quartiles). This assumption can lead to a very rough estimate of the numbers of persons who will need medical care for a succession of illnesses which ultimately culminate in death. The calculations were based on some assumptions regarding the

18. B. N'Galy, S. Bertozzi & R.W. Ryder: 'Obstacles to the optimal management of HIV infection/AIDS in Africa'. *Journal of Acquired Immune Deficiency Syndromes*, 3: 430–7, 1990.

19. C.S. Pandav, K. Anand, B.R. Shamanna, S. Chowdhury & L.M. Nath: 'Economic consequences of HIV/AIDS in India', *Natl Med. J. India*, 10: 27–30, 1997.

TABLE 1: Assumptions of the incidence of HIV infection in India

Age Group	HIV incidence (per thousand)	
	Urban	*Rural*
Newborn	1.5	0.5
15–19	–	–
20–24	5	1.5
25–29	5	1.5
30–34	5	1.5
35–39	2	1
40–44	2	1

Source: Anand et al.

incidence of HIV infection in different age groups in urban and rural populations (Table 1).

Referring back to the original calculations used for the paper cited above, the AIDS-related lifetime mortality expectation can be derived from the calculated incidence of HIV infection as shown in Table 1. Incidence figures are not easy to get and perhaps these assumptions err on the high side. But these are not unlikely values and even if this level has not yet been reached all over the country, it is certain that incidence will touch this level in the not too distant future. If we assume that the prevalence or incidence of the infection has reached a steady state, then the age-specific mortality experience can be taken to be constant for the age groups existing at present. This works out to 289,000 deaths due to AIDS a year in the urban sector and another 283,000 in rural areas (Table 2).

These 572,000 deaths per year are a minimum estimate. If we apply an increment in the incidence of infection, and it is clear that the epidemic is far from mature in India at this time and the number of infected persons is rising rapidly,[20] then many times more will be expected to die from AIDS every year. Applying the

---

20. *National AIDS Control Programme, India. Country Scenario Update*, NACO, MOHFW, p. 12, 1995.

TABLE 2: Projected AIDS deaths in urban and rural India in age group cohorts

Age group of cohort	Year (baseline 1991)	AIDS Deaths Urban (,000)	AIDS Deaths Rural (,000)	Total AIDS Deaths (,000)
0–4	1991–1995	8.2	7.9	16.1
5–9	1996–2000	15.2	16.1	31.3
10–14	2001–2005	14.0	15.0	29.0
15–19	2006–2010	6.9	7.5	14.4
20–24	2011–2015	18.6	16.4	35.0
25–29	2016–2020	41.4	35.5	76.9
30–34	2021–2025	56.0	48.1	104.1
35–39	2026–2030	57.1	53.4	110.5
40–44	2031–2035	39.2	41.6	80.8
45–49	2036–2040	21.5	25.7	47.2
50–54	2041–2045	8.6	12.5	21.2
55–59	2046–2050	2.3	3.3	5.6
60–64	2051–2055	0	0	0
65–69	2056–2060	0	0	0
70 +	2060 +	0	0	0
Total		289.0	283.0	572.0

same logic of six episodes of severe illness including the terminal illness for each person who dies of AIDS, a minimum of 57 million bed days would be required for patients of AIDS annually.

Estimates about the average cost of one bed day varies naturally from hospital to hospital. In the government sector, one bed day at the All India Institute of Medical Sciences (AIIMS) costs Rs 600.[21] Recently the medicine costs of one hospital bed day was calculated to be Rs 250 in a government tertiary care hospital in Bombay.[22] This comes to Rs 160 million annually. In a district hospital on the other hand the cost of one bed for one day comes to only Rs 200.[23] The costs in the private sector

21. P.C. Choubey, Add. Professor of Hospital Administration, All India Institute of Medical Sciences, New Delhi, personal communication, 1997.

22. S.R. Salunke, Director Health Services, Maharashtra, personal communication, 1997.

23. P.C. Choubey, op. cit.

similarly vary greatly but they are in general many times higher than a similar bed / facility in the government sector. Even if we take a figure at the lower end of the range, the 57 million bed days would cost Rs 11,400 million.

Thailand estimates that each person with AIDS costs US $1000 per year in medical expenses not including expensive drugs such as AZT or other anti-HIV drugs.[24] Similarly reports from Malaysia suggest US $2000 per year as the cost of medical care.[25] A report from the Republic of Korea includes AZT and testing and calculates that each patient of AIDS will cost US $4225 in direct medical costs.[26] Even with a minimum estimate of 1.75 million persons infected with HIV in India, the medical costs can be catastrophic for the health system.

Some Implications

It will be noticed that just about half of the cases projected will be in the rural areas. The distribution of hospital beds, however, is unfortunately skewed very heavily towards urban areas. The Ministry of Health and Family Planning reports that of the 596,203 hospital beds in the country, only 122,109 or 20.5 per cent are in the rural areas.[27] This one infection, HIV, has the potential therefore, of requiring 64 per cent of all the hospital beds in the rural area, and for a condition that needs a minimum of Rs 36,000 per patient in direct medical costs. The rural area beds include a large proportion in Primary Health Centres which

---

24. Patrick Giraud: 'The economic impact of AIDS at the sectoral level' in *Economic implications of AIDS in Asia*, D.E. Bloom & J.V. Lyons, UNDP, New Delhi, India. p. 88, 1993.

25. D. Lim: 'Economic impact of AIDS on Malaysia' in *Economic implications of AIDS in Asia*, D.E. Bloom & J.V. Lyons, UNDP, New Delhi, India. p. 63, 1993.

26. Bong-Min Yang: 'The economic impact of AIDS on the Republic of Korea' in *Economic implications of AIDS in Asia*, D.E. Bloom & J.V. Lyons, UNDP, New Delhi, India, p. 50, 1993.

27. Ministry of Health and Family Welfare, *Annual Report, 1995*.

are not, at least as they are at present, adequate to cope with most of the usual opportunistic infections.

There is a marked lack of equity in the provision of health care to rural areas, an imbalance that is not only quantitative in the numbers of beds available, but more importantly a qualitative discrepancy whereby almost every tertiary care and specialist hospital is in the cities. This has resulted in there being a tradition of seeking medical care for serious illnesses in cities rather than in the rural areas. With the increased pressure upon health care facilities in rural areas due to HIV/AIDS, a demand that the existing health care facilities cannot meet, it is inevitable that many of the sick and dying will migrate to the cities to seek help. This will further tax the already overloaded health care facilities in the cities.

In addition, the social welfare infrastructure in the cities will have to cope with the influx of desperately sick people from the rural areas, and their relatives and children. After the patient dies, it is likely that many indigent families will remain as a burden on the city. This tendency will be further augmented by the fact that if the migration to the city to seek help was preceded by a local diagnosis of HIV/AIDS and this has become known, the family may well be social outcasts with nothing to return to. Such a family may prefer to seek the anonymity of a large city.

The Effects upon Mortality

It is logical to conclude that if large numbers of people are going to die of AIDS, there will be an effect upon the mortality indicators in India. It has been feared that in developing countries the gains being made towards reducing infant mortality will be wiped out by the increase due to HIV. Using the model suggested by Stover[28] it is possible to calculate the impact . Table 3 lists the baseline mortality statistics as they are at present in India, and the effect of HIV/AIDS upon them.

---

28. John Stover: 'The impact of HIV/AIDS on adult and child mortality in the developing world', *Health Transition Review*, supplement to vol. 4, 1004, 1994.

TABLE 3: Effect of AIDS upon mortality indicators in India

Indicator	Baseline	Mortality rate revised for AIDS		
		p = 1%	*p = 2.5%*	*p = 5%*
Crude Death Rate	10	10.6	11.4	12.9
Infant Mortality Rate	75	75.6	76.5	78
Under 5 Mortality Rate	110	112.4	115.3	120.7

The effect does not seem to be dramatic. But we must note that all these mortality rates were planned, programmed and expected to go down, in some cases fairly rapidly, during this decade. Yet in every case the potential improvement has been not only halted but reversed. India is entering a period not of steadily declining mortality rates, as the great decade for children so proudly predicted, but of steadily increasing death rates; a step back into the past.

An Agenda for Action: 1. Minimising the Epidemic

It is against this background that the nation has to draw up an agenda for action. In very basic terms two types of plans have to be drawn up and expeditiously implemented: every effort must be made to curb the spread of HIV infection in the country; and the health care system must gird itself to cope with the expected influx of patients with HIV/AIDS-related illnesses.

Curbing the Spread of HIV Infection in the Country

A look at the epidemiology of HIV/AIDS makes it very evident that in India, as in the rest of the world, the spread of the disease in the vast majority of cases is mediated through unprotected sexual contacts. It is estimated that over 85 per cent of new cases of HIV infection can be traced to heterosexual contact.[29] Of the remainder, a significant proportion are in injecting-drug users.

29. NACO: 'Surveillance for HIV Infection/AIDS Cases in India', *Report up to 30 April 1997.*

Infected blood as a source of fresh HIV infection is fortunately rather rare now. Vertical transmission from mother to newborn is likely to assume greater proportions when there is an increase in the number of seropositive pregnant women. HIV/AIDS is a condition which is almost entirely preventable by a combination of behaviour change and attention to blood-mediated spread. The problem lies in ensuring responsible sexual behaviour with safer sex practices whenever in a risk situation.

Understanding of HIV and AIDS

In spite of the fact that awareness programmes based on messages in the electronic media, press and through posters has been going on for quite some time, HIV/AIDS as a conceptualised entity is largely unknown in India. The National Family Health Survey as recently as 1992–93 found that only 36 per cent of ever married women aged 13–49 in Delhi had ever heard about AIDS; in West Bengal and Gujarat only a tiny 10 per cent of the women, and in Maharashtra and Tamil Nadu 19 and 23 per cent respectively of women had heard about AIDS.[30] This is despite the fact that the latter two states are the most affected by the HIV epidemic. Of those who do know, most people when questioned will now be able to say that AIDS is a new disease that is spread through blood and non-sterile syringes. When pressed they will also point out that sex with prostitutes can be the cause of acquiring the infection . Even in Maharashtra and Tamil Nadu 24 and 33 per cent respectively of the women who had heard about AIDS believed that a cure was possible.

Given the very low level of knowledge, even in the states worst hit by the epidemic, and the fact that most people have by and large not experienced AIDS, the incentive to change behaviour is not very strong. Very few persons actually know or have known someone who developed AIDS. The attrition due to

---

30. *National Family Health Survey, Introductory Report,* International Institute for Population Sciences, Bombay, pp. 90–1, Oct. 1994.

AIDS at the workplace, in our communities, within our circle of acquaintances has not made an impact yet.

Ensuring the Safety of the Blood Supply

Efforts are being made to make blood safe though there are reports of blood-mediated HIV infection. Some people have reported that as much as 25 to 75 per cent of blood transfused in this country is not screened.[31] This is probably not true any longer and the actual quantum of unscreened transfusion is probably very much lower.

At present there are an estimated 1114 blood banks in the country; 581 are in the government sector and the remaining 553 are private.[32] According to the December 1995 report from NACO, only 57 per cent of the government blood banks are registered. It is unfortunate that government-owned blood banks constitute a major proportion of the total defaulting units. Fortunately the performance in the private sector is much better with 94 per cent of the blood banks registered and meeting quality standards. Licensed blood banks can be assumed to be taking the precaution of testing blood for HIV antibodies before transfusion. As a result of a public interest litigation by some concerned persons, the Supreme Court has instructed government to ensure that all the blood transfused in the country is tested and safe.[33] Now that the courts have intervened it is likely that all the blood available in blood banks in the country will be screened for HIV.

A concerted effort to educate the medical community of the need to minimise the use of blood has not yet been launched. It must be realised that while the ELISA test for HIV antibodies has a very strong negative predictive value, no test is perfect and a

31. M.K. Jain, T. John & G.T. Keusch: 'A review of human immunodeficiency virus infection in India', *AIDS*, 7: 1185–94, 1994.

32. *National AIDS Control Programme, India. Country Scenario Update.* NACO, MOHFW, p. 68, 1995.

33. Supreme Court of India, Civil Extraordinary Jurisdiction, writ petition (civil) No. 91 of 1992, Common Cause v/s Union of India & Ors.

blood sample in the window period may test negative for HIV antibodies but may be extremely infectious if transfused. Blood must therefore be treated with caution and as a drug. It must be used only when essential. A large number of transfusions are still single unit transfusions. It is well established that there is no medical justification for a single unit transfusion. Lifelines can be kept open by other fluids; transfusion fluids and even plasma expanders are much to be preferred for this purpose.

The usually accepted standard as propagated by the WHO suggests that each hospital bed needs seven units of blood annually. India with 596,203 beds would need more than 4 million units of blood. Rationalisation of blood use has the potential to reduce the demand for blood by 40 per cent, and this will go a long way towards eliminating the need to purchase blood from professional donors. It is professionally donated blood that has the highest risk of being HIV infected.[34] Today nearly 40 per cent of the demand is met from professional donors; thus any reduction in the amount used will reduce a potentially hazardous situation. The goal should be to depend entirely on voluntarily donated blood.

The use of blood components instead of whole blood can also ensure that available blood is used most efficiently and economically. Component separation units need to be made more available and should be a part of every blood bank with a high turnover.

Media Campaigns

A strong media campaign to increase the awareness of HIV/AIDS and propagate condom use is an important part of the activity of NACO. There is still a strong focus on targeted interventions. While targeting HIV/AIDS interventions towards those perceived as being at highest risk is sound health management, it must be kept in mind that those who are at risk today because of their

---

34. J. Hubley, S. Chowdhury & V. Chandramouli: *The AIDS Handbook*, p. 70, 1995.

risk-taking behaviour, may well have been exemplary citizens yesterday, and also may be models of safe behaviour tomorrow. The groups are not static. The large majority of persons in India, probably as in most other countries, have a lifestyle that ensures that they are effectively protected against the possibility of acquiring HIV infection. Some people are at risk. And those at risk have not always been at risk and will not always remain at risk. People move in and out of risk: some changes take place over a long period, others are transient. A well-settled pillar of society, faithful to his wife for many years, may succumb to temptation while out of town or 'drinking with the boys'. The communication strategy must be designed to slow down the movement of persons into the 'at risk' group, and to accelerate the movement of persons whose lifestyle puts them at risk into the behaviour pattern of the vast majority who are protected. Information, Education & Communication (IEC) programmes must have both targeted interventions and mass media components.

Controlling STDs

While HIV/AIDS is an abstract issue to most Indians, even to many decision-makers, STDs are part of our cultural knowledge. In many ways, HIV infection is a sexually transmitted disease. Over 85 per cent of HIV infection is transmitted through the sexual route. It stands to reason that the very measures that are used to prevent STDs in the community also prevent HIV infection. Messages highlighting a new STD, fatal and with no cure, seem to work better than the usual AIDS education. As both STDs and HIV are acquired through the same behaviour and route, they share a common strategy for prevention. The effectiveness of an AIDS awareness and control intervention can be measured by monitoring the trend in prevalence of the conventional STDs, and by measuring changes in behaviour and attitudes.

Scientifically it is now well documented in India[35,36] and in other parts of the world[37,38,39] that the presence of ulcerative genital disease greatly enhances the probability of HIV transmission. A study in Tanzania demonstrated that the treatment of STDs reduced the chance of HIV infection by 42 per cent.[40] Similar results have been reported in other studies.[41] This is perhaps also true of chronic inflammation of the lower reproductive tract. Evidence from studies in Africa suggests that the probability of HIV transmission rises from 1 in 100 to 1 in 20 if genital ulcer disease is present.[42] Even from the limited viewpoint of HIV transmission, it makes good sense to detect STDs as early as possible and treat them rigorously, and to mount an ef-

35. S.M. Mehendale, J.J. Rodrigues, R.S. Brookmeyer, et al.: 'Incidence and predictors of human immunodeficiency virus type I seroconversion in patients attending sexually transmitted disease clinics in India', *J. Infect. Dis.*, 172(6), 1486–91, Dec. 1995.

36. J.J. Rodrigues, S.M. Mehendale, M.F. Shepherd, et al.: 'Risk factors for HIV infection in people attending clinics for sexually transmitted disease in India'. *BMJ*, 29: 311(7000), 283–6, July 1995.

37. I.V. Torian, J.B. Weisfuse, H.A. Makki, D.A. Benson, I.M. DiCamillo & F.F. Toribio: 'Increasing HIV-I seroprevalence associated with genital ulcer disease, New York City, 1990–92', *AIDS* 9(2): 177–81, Feb. 1995.

38. M. Sassan-Morokro, A.F. Greenberg, J.M. Coulibaly, et al.: 'High rates of sexual contact with female sex workers, sexually transmitted disease, and condom neglect among HIV infected and uninfected men with tuberculosis in Abidjan, Cote d'Ivoire', *J. Acquir Immune Defic Syndr Hum Retrovirol.*, 11(2): 183–7, Feb. 1996.

39. F.R. Cleghorn, N. Jack, J.R. Murphy, et al.: 'HIV-I prevalence and risk factors among sexually transmitted disease clinic attenders in Trinidad', *AIDS*, 9(4): 389–94, April 1995.

40. H. Grosskurth, F. Mosha, J. Todd, K. Senkoro, J. Newell, A. Klokke, J. Changalucha, B. West, P. Mayaud, A. Garoyle, R. Gabone, D. Mabey & R. Hayes: 'A Community Trial of the Impact of Improved Sexually Transmitted Disease: The HIV Epidemic in Rural Tanzania—Baseline Survey Results', *AIDS* 9(8): 927–34, 1995.

41. N. O'Farrell: 'Global eradication of donovanosis: an opportunity for limiting the spread of HIV-I infection'. *Genitourin Med.* 71(1): 27–31, Feb. 1995.

42. 'Confronting AIDS: Public Priorities in a Global Epidemic', World Bank Policy Research Report, OUP, New York, 1997.

fective intervention to prevent them. The Government of India now has a strong focus on the treatment of STDs and on reproductive health. If stringently implemented there is every possibility that it will have an important spin-off benefit and tend to restrict the spread of HIV infection.

The management of STDs by using what has come to be known as the 'syndromic approach'[43] has been shown to be effective and is not dependent upon either especial expertise in venereology or on the availability of specialised laboratories. There is an urgent need to propagate the use of the syndromic approach. Using the simple algorithms propagated by WHO can substantially improve the management of such infections. Training in these skills should be made widely available and efforts must be made to develop and propagate similar guidelines for other systems of medicine as well.

Perhaps the most important step would be to influence the treatment-seeking behaviour of persons who contract a sexually transmitted infection. Because of the socio-cultural implications associated with STDs, these persons put very great importance on confidentiality. This, together with the more sympathetic and non-judgmental attitude of non-government health care providers, especially from the traditional systems of medicine, leads a very great proportion of those suffering from such infections to either avoid seeking aid, to procrastinate, or to seek help outside the government system. The Baina study clearly demonstrated the preference for private practitioners over government STD clinics.[44] The latter must be helped to be made more 'user friendly' with a strong focus on maintaining privacy and confidentiality. Unless doctors and the entire staff learn to be non-judgmental, it is unlikely that these clinics will gain wide acceptance.

---

43. *Simplified STD treatment guidelines,* National AIDS Control Organisation, MOHFW, India, 1993.

44. *National AIDS Control Programme, India. Country Scenario Update,* NACO, MOHFW, p. 13, 1995.

Condoms

Even today much of the media advice revolves around the use of condoms. A factor that needs to be kept in mind is the availability of good quality and safe condoms at a price that the poorer people can afford. Using condoms is seen by most people not as an erotic or sensual activity but as a necessary evil. It needs to be made as pleasant a procedure as possible. Good quality, adequately lubricated condoms need to be made easily and widely available. The population must also lose their inhibitions about asking for condoms and education programmes towards these objectives need to be propagated. Mechai in Thailand has shown the way.

Most HIV infection is through unprotected sex with those who have many partners, including sex workers. It is inevitable that these groups are targeted by those planning interventions. Keeping in mind the status of these workers, it is evident that this group is not really empowered to take decisions about patterns of behaviour and the use of personal protective devices such as condoms. It is much more important that the clients of sex workers and the general population are educated. Stigmatising sex workers as the source of infection is not likely to be effective and will certainly ensure their lack of cooperation. Terms such as 'core transmitter groups' should not be used and in any case it seems to put the blame on those marginalised persons who are perhaps more the victims of the scenario rather than the villains. Sex workers themselves can be empowered, however, through a system of peer outreach and collective decision-making insisting on condom use.

It is in this perspective that a communication strategy for behaviour change should be evolved. The messages must necessarily start with the need for an age-related and socially acceptable behaviour strategy. Advocating abstinence, even during youth prior to marriage, is considered old-fashioned and unrealistic. Yet this message not only makes great sense but also has the advantage of being acceptable to a very large segment of our society. Similarly, messages suggesting a mutually faithful relationship between partners need to be stressed.

Sex Education

HIV infection is largely through sex. If it is to be prevented there is no option but to relate its prevention to a responsible and safe sexual lifestyle. The luxury of taking the comfortable and easy way of ignoring sex-related education in our schools and colleges can no longer be afforded. No less a person than Mahatma Gandhi, the Father of the Nation, wrote in favour of sex-related education in schools.[45] Studies in Delhi have shown that senior schoolchildren are very aware of sexual activity amongst their peers. As many as 63 per cent of the boys and 37 per cent of the girls knew of one or more of their peers who were sexually active. The schoolchildren also knew where they could find people willing to have sex with them.[46] In the face of this information, together with reports that the period of maximum sexual experimentation starts upon entering college with its sudden freedom from supervision from both parents and school authorities, it becomes urgent that children are prepared to face the sudden freedom with knowledge and responsibility.

Dr Shankar Chowdhury working with UNESCO introduced the concept of HIV-related education in the school system to decision-makers from countries in the region.[47] In India NCERT has worked with NACO and other resource persons to develop a curriculum that introduces the topic as a part of a gradually evolving adolescence and family life education curriculum in schools.[48] Family life education can be done in a gradually evolv-

45. M.K. Gandhi: As reported in *Hitavada*, 22 January, 1997.
46. S. Chowdhury, P.T. Francis & J.S. Gill: 'Knowledge, beliefs and atttitudes regarding AIDS, STDs and human sexuality among senior secondary students in Delhi', *Indian J. Community Med.*, 19(1): 18, 1994.
47. *Asian region planning Seminar on AIDS education within the school system*, UNESCO, New Delhi, 1994.
48. Seminar report: *Promoting HIV/AIDS Preventive Education within the formal school system in India*, UNESCO, New Delhi, 1997.

ing series that makes children aware of their bodies, prepares them for the changes that take place with growth and development and, when they reach the senior classes, teaches them about responsible sexual behaviour and the dangers of HIV/AIDS.

International Issues

India has a long and relatively permeable land border. In the north-east it borders the golden crescent, and Kashmir is liable to infiltration by mercenaries and terrorists from Pakistan. Both drugs and HIV infection cross into the State of Manipur[49] from Myanmar. It is estimated that there are over 25,000 IV drug users in Manipur and at the last estimate over 77 per cent were already HIV positive.[50] Steps are urgently needed to control the transborder influx of drugs. It is a similar nexus in Kashmir. There is evidence of HIV coming in with terrorists from Pakistan and mercenaries from several nations.

Another issue is the testing of foreigners resident in India. With indigenous cases in the hundreds of thousands if not millions, there is no longer any justification for testing foreigners resident in or visiting India. We have enough HIV of our own and do not need to bother about the occasional visitor who may be living with HIV/AIDS.

Demonstrated Successes

While there is no accepted vaccine against HIV infection as yet, nor a cure for AIDS, there have been many small battles won even as the war against HIV/AIDS continues. Those interventions found successful in other countries should be examined and evaluated for adoption. India has the advantage of getting the infection perhaps ten years later than the West and Africa. We therefore have an opportunity to learn from their successes and

49. S. Sarkar, N. Das, et al.: 'Rapid spread of HIV among injecting drug users in north-eastern states of India', *Bulletin of Narcotics*, 95: 92–105, 1993.

50. AIDS in South East Asia Region, WHO-SEARO, 1998.

avoid the mistakes they made. There is clear evidence that the incidence of HIV infection falls with changes in lifestyle and reduction in risk-taking behaviour. We in India must continue to use all possible avenues of communication to ensure the message of protection against HIV/AIDS gets to all age groups.

The status of women being low results in a woman having no control over her own body. Sex workers cannot normally insist on the client using a condom. But it is not only the sex worker; women in society also have a very low status. In most parts of India it is unthinkable, for example, that a wife should insist that her husband use a condom because she suspects his fidelity. Women's empowerment and economic development will raise their status enough to give them some say about their own lives.

Interventions aimed at establishing 'safe' or 'protected' brothels have shown remarkable results. In Thailand the decline in new infections has been very marked and has been attributed to universal condom use in some brothels.[51] The 'Sonargachi' project in the Calcutta red-light area has demonstrated that such interventions are possible in India also.[52]

Safe injecting practice among injecting-drug users has been shown to be an effective measure against the spread of HIV infection. In Manipur about 70 per cent of injecting-drug users are seropositive. In Australia the figure has been maintained at about 2 per cent.[53] Education about safe injecting works, as does needle exchange or even the inexpensive $2 \times 2 \times 2$ procedure of rinsing the used needle/syringe twice with water, twice with bleach and twice with water again. There is no reason why we cannot teach injecting-drug users to inject safely. The issue of the morality of protecting people from their own folly can be debated endlessly.

---

51. AIDSCAP, Francois-Xavier Bagnoud Centre, Harvard School of Public Health, UNAIDS: *Final Report of the Status and Trends of the Global HIV/AIDS, Pandemic,* July 5–6, 1996.

52. M. Islam, 'AIDS awareness in Sonargachi', *Social Welfare*, 42(8), 23–5, 1995.

53. AIDSCAP, op. cit.

The saving of lives and protecting the spouses of drug addicts cannot wait.

There is now very clear evidence that both the conventional STDs and HIV infection are less probable when the male is circumcised.[54] Studies in Africa have demonstrated that the prevalence of HIV infection is much lower in those peoples who traditionally practise male circumcision.[55] It is time that the message about the advantages of circumcision became more widely known to the general public. It has also been demonstrated that there is a strong correlation between HIV infection and STDs. This is of course due to the fact that both are transmitted by essentially the same route, unprotected sex with infected persons. However, it has also been shown that the presence of ulcerative genital disease, or chronic lower reproductive tract inflammation in itself predisposes to seroconversion in those who are exposed to infection. The inevitable corollary to this is that the early detection and treatment of STDs and other lower reproductive tract infection reduces the chance of getting HIV infection. This must be a prime focus of interventions in India.

An Agenda for Action: 2. Coping with the Increased Demands of the Epidemic Upon the Health System

There are at least 1.75 million persons in the community that have HIV infection; the actual number may be two or even three times greater. All these people are going to fall prey to increasingly severe infections, ultimately culminating in premature death. They are going to need medical care; probably hospital-based care. We must plan today to be able to cope with this

---

54. J. Seed, S. Allen, T. Mertens, et al.: 'Male circumcision, sexually transmitted disease, and risk of HIV', *J. Acquir Immune Def. Syndr. Hum. Retrovirol.*, 8(1): 83–90, Jan. 1995.

55. G.G. Mbugua, L.N. Muthami, C.W. Matura, S.A. Oogo, P.G. Waiyaki, C.P. Lindan & N. Hearst: 'Epidemiology of HIV infection among long distance truck drivers in Kenya', *East Afr Med J*, 72(8): 515–8, Aug. 1995.

expected demand upon the health infrastructure. The issues raised below are merely the outline of a large agenda of very serious, practical matters facing the health system, both public and private. A great deal of energy, expertise and resources needs to be spent on each one, teasing out the details, spelling out the needs, and working on the reality of implementation.

Counselling

With the greatly increased prevalence of HIV infection in the country, there is bound to be a great demand for counselling services. This will not only be a result of increased testing with its attendant pre- and post-test counselling, but also because, as people become more aware of HIV infection and its consequences, they will need advice and support to allay their anxiety and help them cope with the severe mental trauma of being diagnosed as HIV positive. Extreme social, occupational and family crises can be precipitated in HIV positive people and their family and friends. But counselling services are practically non-existent in India and we must start building up the human resources to cope with the inevitable demand. No matter how many counsellors are made available in different health care institutions, there will always be a demand for help and information in a way that ensures privacy and anonymity. A method that has proven of great value in some countries, and is even now meeting a strong need in some parts of India is the telephone helpline or hotline. This is an activity typically run with the help of volunteers but subsidised by government or another donor. This may be one channel that needs to be consciously developed in the urban areas. Perhaps the best persons to run such a service are in the non-government sector. Persons with HIV/AIDS are a useful resource as they can deal with questions with understanding and sensitivity.

Training of Medical and Paramedical Personnel

Human resources in the form of medical personnel, from specialists, other doctors, and nurses to a variety of paraprofes-

sional persons, are involved in modern medical care. The training
and education of the entire team of health care providers must
now have a much greater priority towards HIV-related topics than
hitherto. Undergraduate medical education shows a wide variation in the importance given to HIV as a topic for instruction. We
need to prescribe a standard minimum curriculum to deal with
this topic. Indian medical colleges graduate almost 17,000 new
doctors every year. Unless we take steps expeditiously to include
an approved curriculum on HIV/AIDS in their education, the
backlog of untrained doctors will continue to rise. In addition it is
estimated that there are 4,10,875 registered doctors in India
(1992).[56] While the Indian Medical Association together with
NACO has done yeoman service in running orientation camps for
doctors, there are still thousands of doctors who need training. A
very similar position is true for the 3,85,410 nurses in India.
Curricula need revision and HIV/AIDS needs to be taught to all
levels of health care providers. Considering the fact that there are,
for example, more than 2,03,451 Auxiliary Nurse Midwives
(ANMs) or multipurpose workers (female) in India, as well as
6,09,506 trained dais, this is not a small or simple task.[57]

India has many systems of health care and the practitioners of
these systems provide care to a very substantial number of
people. It is important that all health care providers be adequately
trained to protect themselves and their other patients from HIV
infection. They also need to have the knowledge to recognise the
possibility of HIV/AIDS in their differential diagnoses as they
treat patients. Finally they should be aware of testing, where it
can be done and its fallacies and strengths.

---

56. *Health Information of India*, Central Bureau of Health Intelligence, DGHS,
MOHFW, 1994.

57. Though, as the response to Primary Health Care and the establishment of
community health workers (CHWs) showed in the 70s, political will in
Government can achieve a very great deal.

Universal Precautions

While most large, metropolitan, tertiary care hospitals have some experience by now of dealing with HIV positive individuals and even cases of AIDS, smaller hospitals have not yet had to face this problem in any significant manner. There can be no doubt that these institutions will have to attend to increasing numbers of persons with HIV infection and AIDS. A rigorous programme of training of the staff of such institutions needs to be initiated, together with a continuing education process, to increase their skills in handling HIV/AIDS. A similar situation exists in the case of private practitioners.

It must be emphasised that, in general, care-givers, including hospital staff and family members, are not at risk from the HIV/AIDS patients that they look after.[58] Even needle stick injuries with a known HIV positive element have been shown to have a seroconversion rate of less than 1 in 1000.[59] Providers of health care need the knowledge and skill to protect themselves from HIV and its consequences. For example, those handling an opportunistic infection such as Koch's, especially disseminated Koch's infection, need to wear masks. This is not to protect themselves against HIV, but to protect themselves against tuberculosis. Laboratory staff also need to be constantly reminded that they are dealing with potentially infectious material and to make use of all prescribed, personal, protective devices such as masks and eye shields. A group that has a very particular need of skill augmentation in this area are dentists. They are perhaps amongst those health care providers who are at highest risk.

Most hospitals are not yet taking 'Universal Precautions' very seriously even in the large tertiary care institutions. A recent

58. B. N'Galy, R.W. Ryder, K. Bila, et al.: 'Human Immunodeficiency Virus infection among employees in an African Hospital', *New England J Med*, 319(7): 1123–7, 1988.

59. Torkars, J.I. et al., 'For the CDC Cooperative Needle-stick Surveillance of HIV Infection and Zidovudine use Amongst Healthcare Workers after Exposure to HIV Infected Blood', *Ann. Intern. Med.,* 118: 913–19, 1993.

study in Delhi showed many lacunae even in one of the most prestigious institutions in the country.[60] The medical fraternity needs to make sure these precautions are taken so that both the patient and the health care provider are protected. There is a role here for institutions such as the Medical Council of India, the Indian Medical Association, the Association of Hospital Administrators, the Indian Association of Preventive and Social Medicine, the National Academy and the like.

Primary Health Care

As pointed out earlier, there is a marked lack of equity in the rural/urban division of health care resources. While 70 per cent of the population lives in rural areas, more than 70 per cent of health expenditure is in urban areas. With the onset of HIV/AIDS, rural health care facilities will have to be built up. As AIDS becomes commonplace, we will have no alternative to well-supported home-based care, and this support will have to come from primary and secondary care institutions.

In addition, while the treatment of some of the infections associated with HIV/AIDS would normally be expected to be done at the tertiary or at the least at the district or secondary care hospitals, the sheer pressure of numbers will result in many cases being handled by the Primary Health Centre (PHC). This has implications not only for training but also for augmenting the resources available at the PHC. Even secondary care institutions such as district hospitals are not yet geared to adequately cope with HIV/AIDS. It is vital, for example, that the drugs needed for treating the more common opportunistic infections are made available; also gloves, disposable needles, and the other materials and equipment necessary to protect staff and patients from infection. As HIV/AIDS starts manifesting more frequently in the rural areas this training and the provision of drugs and resources will

---

60. R. Kucheria: 'A hospital based study of knowledge and practices of health care workers regarding Universal Precautions against HIV', Thesis for MD, All India Institute of Medical Sciences, New Delhi, 1996.

have to be made available in Primary Health Centres. As there are 2,242 Community Health Centres, 21,853 Primary Health Centres, and 1,32,727 Subcentres in India (as of 31 March 1996[61]), this will be no small undertaking.

Tuberculosis

Tuberculosis is one of the infections most frequently associated with HIV infection and compromised immunity.[62] Reports from India and Nepal state that 83 and 75 per cent of AIDS patients develop tuberculosis.[63,64] So common is tuberculosis in HIV positive persons that in several parts of the world it has become an accepted practice to put persons found to be HIV positive on routine anti-tubercular therapy. With the increased prevalence of HIV infection, there is likely to be a steady increase in the number of persons needing anti-tubercular therapy. In anticipation, it seems prudent to strengthen the diagnostic and therapeutic infrastructure for managing patients with tuberculosis. Unlike HIV, tuberculosis is a hazard to health care providers, including those at home.

It is reported that there are over 14 million persons with active tuberculosis in India.[65] With the advent of HIV infection this number is likely to increase significantly. Fortunately directly observed treatment (DOT) holds out a promise of effective management. A completed course of treatment with the several drugs prescribed helps not only to cure the patient but also prevents the emergence of resistant strains. In some parts of the

---

61. *Annual Report 1996–97*, Ministry of Health and Family Welfare, Government of India, p. 33.

62. A.D. Arries: 'Tuberculosis and Human Immunodeficiency Virus infection in developing countries'. *Lancet,* 335: 387–90, 1990.

63. J. Narain: 'HIV and Tuberculosis Surveillance: An overview or programmatic issues', in *Roundtable on HIV/AIDS Surveillance in India*, 1997.

64. D.N. Lanjewar & V.L. Wagholikar: 'Mycobacteriosis emerges as most common infection in AIDS victims of India', *VIII International Conference on AIDS/III World STD Congress*, Amsterdam, July 1992. (Abstract PoB3556)

65. *Annual Report*, MOHFW, p. 167, 1996–97.

world forms of tuberculosis resistant to multiple drugs have become an important problem. We have to be prepared for MDR and those treating tuberculosis must have a high index of suspicion in this regard.

Home Care

There is no way that we can mobilise enough beds to hospitalise all those persons with HIV infection needing extra care due to a concomitant infection. India must start preparing for home care. An attitude has to be built up, first amongst health care providers, and then, through them amongst people with HIV infection and their families: an attitude and understanding that most people with AIDS can be looked after adequately at home for most of the time. This not only saves hospital resources for the critically ill, but ensures that the patient is treated humanely and with the help and support of his/her loved ones.

Home care as a concept does not mean leaving the person needing care unattended to live or die in his/her home. The health system must plan to meet the special needs that make home care possible, and ensure support for the appropriate way of looking after patients with AIDS.[66] First and foremost is the training that the family will need; this can be provided by a well-prepared health visitor or public health nurse.[67] This category of health staff will have to be trained and given the skills needed for communicating with and supporting families trying to come to grips with a seriously ill loved one, frequently the breadwinner. Second, both professional staff and volunteers will have to be available to support the family and the patient in his/her medical needs. It is critical that essential drugs are available at this level. This coordinated approach will be expensive to establish; but it should not be beyond the reach of the poor.

---

66. V.H. Raveiss & K. Siegal: 'The impact of care giving on informal or familial care givers', *AIDS Patient Care*, 39–43, 1991.
67. D. Ward & M.A. Brown: 'Labor and costs in AIDS family caregiving', *Western J Nursing Research*, 16: 10–22, 1994.

Social and Welfare Problems

One of the many non-medical problems associated with this disease is the lack of income and financial support for the family in time of crisis. This has tremendous repercussions on every aspect of the life of the entire family. Fortunately the HIV-infected person has a fairly long time of reasonable health when he or she can continue to work and support his or her family. HIV positive persons need help in making provisions for their illness and the family thereafter. Some form of social security or health insurance should be established to meet this need. For those who are, or become, indigent, government may have to invest in a scheme to support them and their families.

Of particular importance are the needs of children. 'AIDS orphans'[68] are one of the more depressing and dreadful consequences of this disease. Provisions will have to be made for the welfare, education and foster care of increasing numbers of orphans. One estimate made in Lusaka suggested that 10 per cent of the children in the capital of Zambia had lost one or both of their parents.[69] It has been estimated that by 1995 there were 3.7 million AIDS orphans in the world.[70] In India too, when AIDS deaths become very common, hundreds of thousands of children are likely to lose one, or frequently both, of their parents. This has to be planned for and a policy regarding state responsibility decided. It would be advisable to encourage mechanisms for community support. Besides the consequences that children would have to face by being deprived of parental support, there is also the problem of children who become infected with the virus. Dr Jonathan Mann had estimated that by 1995 there would be 14,94,900 children in the world infected with AIDS.[71] India will have to bear her share of this dreadful toll.

---

68. D. Michaels & C. Levine: 'Estimates of the number of motherless youth orphaned by AIDS in the United States', *JAMA*, 268: 3456–61, 1992.

69. K.S. Baboo: Prof. of Preventive Medicine, University Teaching Hospital, Lusaka, Zambia, personal communication, 1991.

70. J. Mann: Quoted in brochure of the Association Francois-Xavier Bagnoud.

71. J. Mann: in *AIDS in the World*, OUP, 1992.

Terminal Care

While home care can take much of the load from the hospital without compromising the care of patients, families and communities will need help in dealing with terminally ill patients. The models that have proven of some benefit in other countries are the hospices run by charitable and religious organisations, and terminal care facilities as distinct from hospitals. It is important that such facilities are established widely, starting in those metropolitan areas where HIV/AIDS is already taking its grim toll.

Budget and Drug Supply

The scenario as it appears at present indicates that the health system will have to augment its budget to cope with the increased demands by people with HIV/AIDS. Unless such projections and demands are made to the authorities responsible for budget allocations from now on, it may be impossible to cope with the influx of patients.

The treatment of HIV/AIDS is evolving from day to day. A very significant breakthrough was made with the advent of anti-retroviral therapy, particularly the triple combination treatment. This therapeutic regime holds out the promise of prolonging life, reducing opportunistic infections, and even the hope that eventually HIV/AIDS will be viewed as a chronic infection requiring outpatient management. However that is in the future. Today the triple therapy is very expensive, costing about US $1500 per month per patient.[72] Besides cost, there are problems associated with monitoring, follow-up care and support, and maintaining drug availability. Neither the cost, the availability of the monitoring and support system, nor even the availability of the drug are conducive to the triple regime being available to general patients in developing countries. The public health system at the moment

---

72. WHO Press Release WHO/37, 29 April, 1997.

may have no choice but to restrict their pharmacopoeia to the drugs used for treating the usual opportunistic infections. However, as discussed above, even this latter restricted drug availability will put an unbearable strain on the resources available to the health system.

But there is one new therapy that should be considered by the public health system. It has been shown that the new treatments can cut down the risk of peri-natal transmission of HIV infection by 70 per cent;[73] and even AZT will halve the chances of the newborn being infected. AZT is not as expensive as the anti-retrovirals and was once available in India at a very reasonable price. The public health system should consider making AZT available to pregnant women who are seropositive. The cost effectiveness of this step may make it worthwhile.

Conclusions

There are a great many people in India who are already infected with HIV. It is likely that the number is somewhere between 1.5 and 4.5 million. While we cannot say precisely what it is, it is certain that even with the most conservative estimate, the number is large enough to constitute a social, economic and public health disaster that threatens many of the welfare systems of the country. As far as the current state of knowledge of this disease allows us to predict, virtually all these persons will either eventually develop clinical AIDS and die, or, earlier, succumb to an infection resulting from their diminished immune system. This will leave many indigent families and orphans who will become the state's responsibility and a state liability. For those infected, even more than the final terminal event, the repeated episodes of sickness that is a part of HIV disease, and that each is likely to undergo, will be a burden upon the health system. The demands

---

73. WHO Fact Sheet No 163, May 1997.

upon the health care infrastructure are likely to be of a magnitude that could well cause the system to collapse.

The nation urgently needs to take steps to prevent, as far as possible, the spread of HIV infection, and to plan for meeting the inevitable deluge of patients needing medical, nutritional, psychological, economic and social care. Health promotion and the conscious preservation of traditionally accepted norms promoting responsible sexual behaviour are required. Human resources need to be built up, and budgets augmented manifold. Equally urgently necessary are well-planned and deliberate steps to energise social and community mechanisms to take the responsibility for a part of the burden. Practitioners of other systems of medicine need to be informed and actively involved in programmes against HIV/AIDS.

The fight against HIV/AIDS cannot be won by government health systems alone, no matter how enlightened and efficient their approach. The community, NGOs and the private health sector must all play a role. Persons with HIV/AIDS, CSWs and other groups directly involved should also be a part of the strategic planning and decision-making process.

Together against AIDS we can still make a better future.

* * *

Discussion: The Personal Face of the Epidemic

PG: Dr Nath has described some of the ways the health system needs to respond to the epidemic. From your own experience, are there specific aspects of this that you think need emphasis?

S: 'Ideally, care for people with HIV disease includes a broad range of health care and social services designed to enhance the quality of life, maximise individual choice and minimise hospital and institutional care. Such services should be rendered with compassion in a manner that allows people with HIV disease and their loved ones to act as partners with their care-givers.' That is a quote from somewhere; I can't remember where. But it is quite right. That is the specific response needed from the health system, for people with HIV disease.

PG: It sounds a bit like something from the UN; rather vague and general. What does it mean in specifics?

S: As a person with HIV, and one who has had the privilege of meeting hundreds of people with HIV across the country, I have been able to document a number of elements indispensable for delivering continuous and comprehensive services for people with HIV infection. These include:

- HIV antibody testing that is voluntary and must be accompanied by counselling; both anonymous (unlinked) and confidential testing contribute in different ways, and both options should be available.
- Medical services for PLWHA require a multidisciplinary care approach in which a team of health care providers—including primary care physicians and consultants in other specialities, nutritionists, psychologists and mental health specialists, work together with PLWHA and their families.
- A range of services for PLWHA, from minor help for PLWHA living at home, to congregate living facilities with support services, to skilled nursing and specialist medical care.

As the number of PLWHA grows, the availability of health care professionals experienced and knowledgeable in dealing with HIV is an increasing concern. HIV education and training programmes for better health care delivery must be improved and expanded.

PG: I think it is also important to talk not just about the need for services to be provided, but also the part we can all play in defining and determining what form those services will take. As 'Positive Life', a group of people directly affected by the epidemic, either themselves or through their families and loved ones, puts it: 'We wish to bring home the truth that HIV affects not only those living with it, but many others around them, who also need to be addressed and included.... In this way we hope more and more people directly affected and living with HIV will have access to and will also network for services that they need. This will create a high level of involvement of this community as the end users of the services and hence, place them in positions of decision-making and empowered self-care.'

'Positive Life' also suggests that the kinds of 'services' needed are more than simple health care. As their Mission Statement says: 'We, at Positive Life believe that HIV needs a holistic continuum of care for those living with HIV, as well as the affected. We strive for (a) the wholesome involvement of the infected and affected community with capacity enhancement, participatory decision-making and empowered self-care; (b) the creation of a "safe" platform for any affected people to network—with no pressures or threats of exposure of identities; and (c) the formation and execution of an effective resource-service-advocacy network.'

Changes in Mortality in Mumbai: Monitoring Mortality to Analyse the Spread of HIV

EMMANUEL ELIOT

The actual number of people who are HIV positive in India is not known. Between 1986 and February 1998 the nationwide surveillance system reported 73,481 HIV positive and 5,181 AIDS cases.[1] The north-eastern States (Manipur and Nagaland) as well as Maharashtra and Goa have reported the highest proportion of seropositive cases. But these data are dependent upon the testing capacity of each State, and are accepted to be widely under-reported: some States do not test people regularly and do not send the results to the Central Government. Moreover, these data are biased by a high proportion of tests being from 'high-risk groups' and by an over-representation of patients at government hospitals. Thus, besides this lack of knowledge about the real number of HIV positive cases, these statistics do not allow us to analyse the demographic implications of the epidemic, nor to prepare action programmes.

The main demographic implication is the impact on mortality the HIV epidemic must have.[2] Some diseases have a strong link

---

1. *Monthly update of HIV infection in India:* NACO, Ministry of Health and Family Welfare, Government of India, 28 February 1998.

2. See, for example, B. Cohen & James Trussel, eds., *Preventing and Mitigating AIDS in Sub-Saharan Africa*, National Academy Press, Washington DC, 1996; Michel Garenne et al., 'Mortality Impact of AIDS in Abidjan, 1986–1992', *AIDS 1996*, 10:1279–86; Alan Whiteside and John Stover, 'The Demographic and Economic Impact of AIDS in Africa', *AIDS 1997*, 11(suppl. B): 555–61.

with HIV, like tuberculosis; such diseases will increase in particular age groups, and, in particular, young adults will die earlier. Monitoring mortality could thus be a good indicator of the spread of the HIV epidemic, while waiting for the diagnostics and statistics of HIV itself to improve. The aim of this chapter is to analyse the mortality and the causes of death in Brihan Mumbai (Greater Bombay) from a geographic and demographic point of view.

The Study

The Location: Brihan Mumbai (Greater Bombay)

Mumbai, the capital of Maharasthra State, is the second most populated city of India with 9.9 million inhabitants, according to the latest census (1991). It is the main economic centre of the country and welcomes, because of its status, migrant workers from all over India, especially from Uttar Pradesh and Bihar. Space is the major problem for this city which, being a peninsula, is limited by its natural boundaries. In 1991, the density was 16,432 persons per square kilometre, a level of crowding which generates problems of pollution, congestion and housing.

Brihan Mumbai is also known as the 'AIDS capital' of India. It was one of the first cities in India to establish HIV testing facilities, in 1996. This might explain the high number of reported cases of HIV. In Maharashtra, the HIV seroprevalence map is based on data collected at the State Directorate of Health Services. It presents the number of HIV positive cases for all the groups tested per district. The categories of risk factor/group are the following: heterosexuals (128 per thousand), intravenous drug users (62 per thousand), blood donors and recipients of blood products (36 per thousand), antenatal mothers (10 per thousand), others (103 per thousand).[3]

---

3. Directorate of Health Services: *An overview of the HIV/AIDS problem in Maharashtra State*, 30 June 1995.

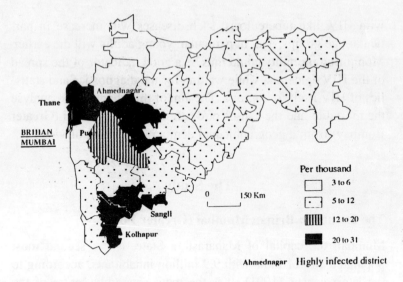

FIGURE 1: HIV prevalence in 1995 in Maharashtra State (Districtwise).

By 1995, HIV infection had spread throughout Maharashtra (Figure 1) with the urban districts of Pune and Mumbai having high HIV prevalence (12 to 20 per thousand).[4] The industrial peripheries of Thane and Ahmednagar, however, as well as the two districts of Kolhapur and Sangli, which are communication centres to Karnataka, reported even higher seroprevalence (between 21 and 31 per thousand).

The Data Sources

1. *Mortality data* from the Mumbai Municipal Corporation (MMC) where statistics for the years 1986[5]/1989/1991/1994 have been collected.[6] Three-year periods have been chosen for a more homogeneous sample. The 1986 and 1989 information comes

---

4.   Government of Maharashtra, Directorate of Health Services: *ZBTCwise, yearwise blood samples screening and positivity.*.

5.   Date of the first AIDS and HIV detected cases in India.

6.   I am thankful to Dr Salunke Director, Directorate of Health Services, Maharashtra as well as Dr Alka Karhande, Executive Health Officer, Mumbai Municipal Corporation and her staff.

from the Annual Reports of the Executive Health Office. For the years 1991 and 1994, the data have been collected by the author. Two particular aspects of these data were focused upon: number of deaths and their causes, which are available for each ward for some particular diseases; and deaths by age group and sex for each collected year. The quality of these data is high because the death registration system is efficient in Brihan Mumbai. In a system quite possibly unique to India, and largely arising from the vast population size and high urban growth, a death certificate from a doctor or health officer is required for each cremation or burial. The death is declared at the place of residence. For the poorest part of the population that cannot afford to pay, five signatures of the family or relatives are required; this is called 'Panchanama'. This death registration system is widely reported to be efficient, and has been in place for many years. Thus, any changes in death rates in the metropolis are unlikely to be the result of a recent improvement in reporting. Unfortunately, the causes of death by age groups were not available for the year 1994 during the enquiry.

2. *Population data* from the Census of India 1981 and 1991, especially the population totals of each ward; and projections made by the author for the years 1986, 1989 and 1994.

3. *HIV seroprevalence data* collected during the period 1988 and May 1994 in Brihan Mumbai hospitals:[7] most of them belong to the central parts of the city although two were situated in the north west. This geographical distribution, as well as a high proportion of government hospitals included in the group from which data were collected imply that this is by no means a statistically representative sample. It is currently, however, the best available data on HIV prevalence in Mumbai and is highly suggestive.

---

7. S. Bharat, *Facing the Challenge: household and community response to HIV/AIDS in Mumbai, India,* World Health Organisation, Geneva, 1996.
I am very thankful to Mrs Bharat (reader at the Tata Institute of Social Sciences) for her help and her discussions about the study in Brihan Mumbai.

The variation in the time periods between the first two sets of data and the arbitrary nature of the HIV data might cause some criticism of this analysis. The response to this is that the present study uses the best data available, and suggests trends which can and should be verified using more detailed and sophisticated data collection.

An Increase in Mortality in Brihan Mumbai

The Trend in Brihan Mumbai

Between the years 1986 and 1994 overall mortality increased in Mumbai by 6 per cent. This increase in mortality is variable according to the age groups and through the years (Figure 2). Looking at the actual numbers of deaths in Mumbai during this period, the graph reveals four trends:

- A general decrease in death for the youngest age groups, especially since 1991. This could be due to an improvement of health status of this age group, resulting from strengthened health programmes, care and services.
- An increase since 1986 in the number of deaths among prime-age adults.
- An increase in deaths among teenagers since 1991.
- A decrease in deaths since 1991 among the oldest age-groups.

Thus, 1991 seems to mark a transition between two patterns of mortality. However, this increase in mortality could be linked with the population growth of the Maharashtrian metropolis, which, for the period 1981 to 1991 was 18.99 per cent. To establish whether this increase in mortality was linked with the population growth over this period a set of age-specific mortality rates was constructed for the years 1986, 1989, 1991 and 1994 (Table 1). These show a significant net increase in mortality in Mumbai for several age groups (Figures 3 and 4). Specifically:

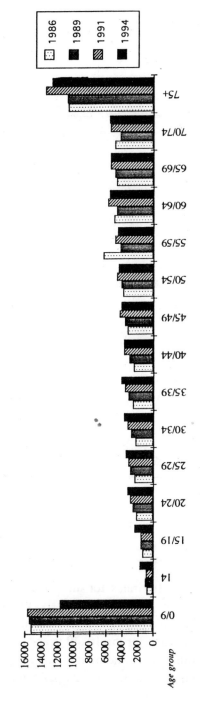

FIGURE 2: Number of deaths 1986/1989/1991/1994 in Brihan Mumbai.

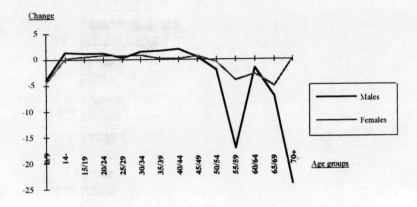

FIGURE 3: Change in age-specific mortality rates (1986/1994) in Mumbai.

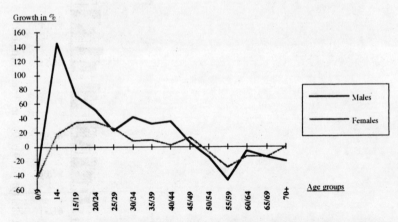

FIGURE 4: Percent change in age specific mortality rates (1986/1994) in Mumbai.

- Mortality rates for all Brihan Mumbai increased for the age group 10–49 years: nearly 150 per cent increase for 10–14 year-old boys and a substantial increase for the 15–49 year-old men and for the 10–49 year-old women.
- Infant and child mortality, however, has fallen in Mumbai over this period by some 25 per cent.

TABLE 1: Age-specific mortality rates in Brihan Mumbai

Age Group	Death rates per 1000: 1986		
	Male	Female	Total
0–9 years	10.1	10.21	10.15
10–14 years	0.95	0.78	0.87
15–19 years	1.65	1.5	1.58
20–24 years	2.21	2.07	2.15
25–29 years	2.86	2.14	2.5
30–34 years	3.6	2.33	2.47
35–39 years	4.93	2.4	3.07
40–44 years	5.64	3.35	4.73
45–49 years	9.36	4.77	7.48
50–54 years	13.9	7.8	11.5
55–59 years	36.8	14.36	27.53
60–64 years	29.94	20.43	25.82
65–69 years	50.31	36.8	43.92
70+ years	114.93	99.93	107.16

Age group	Death rates per 1000: 1989		
	Male	Female	Total
0–9 years	8.53	8.99	8.76
10–14 years	1.04	1.07	1.06
15–19 years	1.81	1.7	1.76
20–24 years	2.64	3.5	3.01
25–29 years	3.4	2.32	2.91
30–34 years	4.3	2.3	3.45
35–39 years	5.44	2.94	4.19
40–44 years	6.47	3.82	5.15
45–49 years	9.78	5.36	7.95
50–54 years	14.43	7.37	11.56
55–59 years	21.18	11.52	17.06
60–64 years	28.37	17.69	23.45
65–69 years	46.94	33.84	40.78
70+ years	91.08	94.51	92.82

TABLE 1: Contd

Age group	Death rates per 1000: 1991		
	Male	Female	Total
0–9 years	8.16	7.95	8.06
10–14 years	0.91	0.98	0.95
15–19 years	1.83	1.66	1.75
20–24 years	2.9	2.4	2.69
25–29 years	3.6	2.5	3.1
30–34 years	4.7	1.87	3.76
35–39 years	7.7	2.8	4.72
40–44 years	8	3.8	6.28
45–49 years	9.9	7.2	6.24
50–54 years	15.9	7.2	12.36
55–59 years	23.61	11.55	17.58
60–64 years	33.4	19.07	26.24
65–69 years	50.13	33.68	41.91
70+ years	108.82	108.7	108.7

Age group	Death rates per 1000: 1994		
	Male	Female	Total
0–9 years	6.03	5.65	5.85
10–14 years	2.33	0.92	1.63
15–19 years	2.83	2.01	2.46
20–24 years	3.36	2.88	3.1
25–29 years	3.5	2.7	3.14
30–34 years	5.09	2.51	3.97
35–39 years	8.5	2.62	4.78
40–44 years	7.68	3.41	5.91
45–49 years	9.9	5.4	8.05
50–54 years	11.92	7.2	9.94
55–59 years	19.64	10.27	15.43
60–64 years	28.22	17.67	23.32
65–69 years	43.22	31.68	37.9
70+ years	90.96	100.13	94.14

- The oldest age groups also experienced a very significant decrease in mortality—nearly 75 per cent among the oldest groups. This suggests the 'greying' of Mumbai: the increase in an ageing population.
- The increase in mortality was higher for males than for females: + 13.72 and + 11.70 per cent respectively for the whole period.

The graphs show three main features; that infant and child mortality has gone down; that younger, prime-age adults are dying in larger numbers than would be expected; and that older adults are surviving longer. The second of these is the central issue in this chapter.

Figure 5 divides the increase in the mortality rates between 1986–89 and 1991–94. Strikingly, the greatest increases in mortality occur after 1991.

While it is accepted that these data show no direct connection between mortality and HIV, it is strongly suggested that this increase in mortality is the result of the wide spread of HIV infection among the population of Brihan Mumbai during the last ten years. This increase in mortality among young adults is exactly

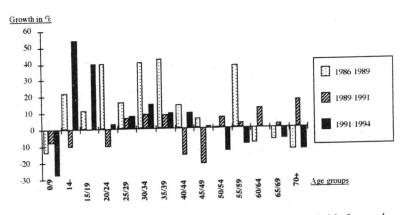

FIGURE 5: Percent change in age-specific mortality rates in Mumbai before and after 1991.

what one would expect with the prevalence of HIV that is estimated for Mumbai, and there does not appear to be any apparent alternative cause for it. An extremely unexpected finding, however, is the fact that the greatest increase in mortality is among boys of 10 to 14 years. If this increase in mortality is related to HIV, two important points need to be made: first, that this means that boys are becoming infected at a very early age, quite possibly at or before 10 years of age; and secondly that it suggests an aspect of the epidemic (the spread of HIV among young boys) to which very little attention has so far been paid, and for which very few responses are in place.

Mortality Increases at Ward Level

The ward level data[8] were also examined. Unfortunately it was not possible to determine age-specific mortality rates by ward; however, the population growth problem was dealt with by comparing the ward level percentage increase in mortality with the percentage increase in population between 1986 and 1994. Two groups of wards (Figure 6) can be distinguished. On the one hand, wards where population growth was greater than the increase in mortality (group 2)—wards where the increase in mortality was linked with and probably resulted largely from in-migration and consequent population growth. On the other hand, there were nine wards where the increase in mortality did not seem to be linked with the arrival of new inhabitants (group 1). These particular areas seem to have experienced 'abnormal mortality' for this period. There is no particular trend in their spatial distribution in Brihan Mumbai, although the northern and central parts of the city mainly belong to this first group.

An example will make this clear. In ward E, which is near the congested heart of the peninsula, the population grew by 2.6 per cent during the period 1981–91; but the overall mortality increased between 1986 and 1994 in that ward by 10.6 per cent. The problem of the lack of complete time-overlap of the two data

---

8.   Brihan Mumbai is divided into 23 wards.

sets referred to above is made clear by this example. Unofficial, professional estimates, however, are clear that there is unlikely to have been any major change in population growth patterns in Mumbai between 1991 and 1994.

The connections between population growth and mortality increase are complex; where population growth is the result of natural increase, mortality itself would be expected to increase at the same rate as the population, unless there was a significant change in the health status of that population.[9] If the population growth is largely a result of in-migration, an increase in mortality will tend to reflect the age-specific mortality rates of the migrants. Most migrants to Mumbai are prime-age adults, whose age-specific mortality rates are very low (an average of 0.2 per cent for Mumbai, for instance). From the present data, the increases in mortality are generally clearly on a much larger scale and are greater than the increases in population, signifying substantial changes in mortality rates in those wards. Even in many of the wards where population growth is higher than the increase in mortality, and is so high as to be clearly *not* the result of natural increase, but obviously a result of in-migration (e.g. wards R-north, M-east, K-west and R-south), the increases in mortality are very much greater than would be expected, given what has been said about the probable age-specific mortality rates of the likely migrants.

The Epidemiological Transition Model

At the beginning of the 1970s, Omram[10] created a new model of health status analysis based on the demographic transition model.

---

9. That is, the mortality rates would not change, so an addition of *x* number of people within a year (or *y*% of the previous year's population) would see an additional *z* deaths (or *y*%—the same proportion as the population increase—of previous annual deaths). If the health status of the population improves, mortality rates will go down; then both numbers of deaths, and percentage of previous annual deaths—and of any population increase—will decrease.

10. A.R. Omran, 'The epidemiological transition: a theory of the epidemiology of population change', *Milbank Fund Quarterly,* 49, No. 1, pp. 509–38, 1971.

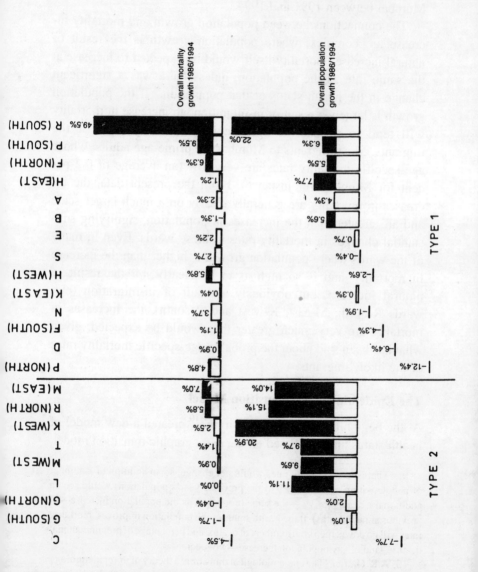

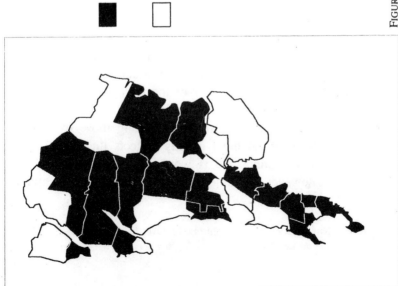

TYPE 1: Mortality increase **above** the population growth

TYPE 2: Mortality growth **below** the population growth

FIGURE. 6: Two groups of wards in Mumbai.

The aim of his analysis was to understand the spatial as well as social disparities of death. For a long time, infectious and parasitic diseases constituted the main causes of death. With the increase in the age of death, new types of diseases appeared: heart disease, cancer, diabetes, etc,. as well as diseases created by human beings like accidents at work and those caused by pollution.

There is thus a strong relationship between economic as well as social development and the epidemiological transition model. In western countries, most people die old and the main causes of death are cardiovascular diseases, tumours, etc. In developing countries, city dwellers run a dual risk: they are still affected by infectious and parasitic diseases as well as 'new diseases' (cancer and heart diseases).

The World Bank, in a seminal book,[11] made this model the basis for a serious look at health policy. The authors identify the increase in absolute numbers of older adults, as well as an increase in the proportion of older adults in the population, as the basis of the health transition. The consequences are the need for increasingly expensive medical services for increasing numbers of older people.

The two age pyramids (Figure 7) confirm what has been revealed earlier. In ten years (1981–1991), we can note a tightening around the adults but more especially around the oldest age groups. However, the high number of the youngest age groups (0–9 years) is still the sign of a developing country.

The dramatic decrease in mortality among those over 50 during this decade in Mumbai exactly reflects this health or epidemiological transition, and is worth separate study on its own. It is not, however, the subject of this chapter, except insofar

11. R. Feacham, T. Kiellstrom, C. Murray, M. Over & M. Phillips, eds: '*The health of adults in the developing world*', OUP, New York, 1992.

as it highlights the 'abnormality' of the increase in prime-age adult mortality that has occurred in Mumbai.

Causes of Death in Brihan Mumbai

Although no data were available regarding the causes of death by age group for the period studied (1986–94), it is interesting to see whether there are any particular trends in the cause of death in Brihan Mumbai.

An Analysis of Seven Main Causes of Death

Seven groups have been selected for the analysis—cancer neoplasms, heart diseases, pulmonary diseases (excluding tuberculosis), tuberculosis (TB), diarrhoea, hepatitis, and 'other diseases'. This last group includes all the viral diseases (tropical or otherwise), transport and domestic accidents, diseases of the female gynaecological system as well as deaths under enquiry.

Of these selected groups representing the main causes of death, heart diseases, cancer, pulmonary disease, TB, diarrhoea and hepatitis accounted for 56.7 per cent of the total causes of death in 1986. Hepatitis, tuberculosis and diarrhoea are especially well known for their interaction with HIV.

A study between 1987 and 1993 of 100 symptomatic HIV positive patients[12] (most of them with multiple opportunistic infections) in Chennai (Madras) revealed that tuberculosis was the most common opportunistic disease (36.7 per cent of the total), followed by oral candidiasis (24.6 per cent) and diarrhoea (14.4 per cent). The other opportunistic infections noted were herpes zoster, cryptococcal meningitis, and fungal infection of the skin, but these represented a small proportion.

---

12. Kumarasamy, N. et al.: 'Spectrum of opportunistic infections among AIDS patients in Tamil Nadu, India', *International Journal of STD and AIDS*, Volume 6: 447–9, 1995.

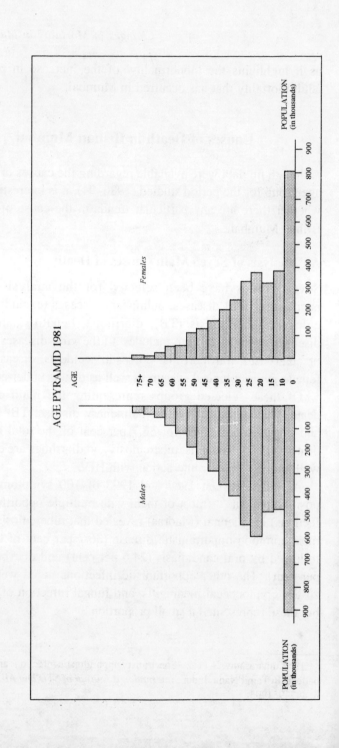

AGE PYRAMID 1981

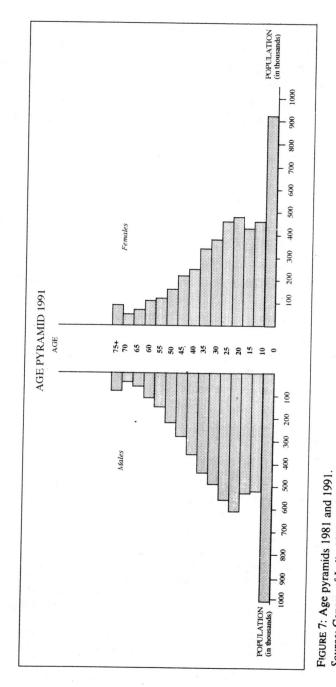

FIGURE 7: Age pyramids 1981 and 1991.
Source: Census of India 1981 and 1991.

The HIV/TB link is very dangerous. The World Health Organisation estimated in 1990 that over 75 per cent of the 1.7 billion people globally infected with TB lived in developing countries. India is one of the most infected countries in the world. TB has long been endemic and its incidence is increasing today. Another study in Chennai on 1,430 TB patients[13] revealed that HIV seropositivity rose from 0.77 per cent in 1991 to 3.4 per cent in 1993. It also showed that TB patients with HIV infection were in the early phase of immunosuppression.

Regarding hepatitis[14], a study at the Christian Medical College, Vellore (Tamil Nadu) on 35,395 blood donors between 1986 and 1988 showed that approximately 2 per cent of the patients had dual infection (HIV and hepatitis B).

Diarrhoea is a common disease in developing countries and a marker of HIV; thus, high increases could reveal some abnormal trends.

In fact, these three diseases could constitute indicators of the spread of HIV until the testing system improves. It may be suggested that sexually transmitted diseases could have been included in this group; unfortunately, data were not available. Also, cancer has not been selected as an important cause of death due to HIV in this study for one particular reason: Kaposi's sarcoma—one of the main tumours in AIDS patients—seems to be rare in Indians.[15]

The analysis of changes in occurrence of these causes of death in Mumbai reveals an increase for all, except for diarrhoea, deaths from which declined by 30.16 per cent over the period 1986–94. The highest increase was for hepatitis (+247 per cent),

---

13. Solomon, S. et al.: 'Trend of HIV infection in patients with pulmonary tuberculosis in South India', *Tubercle and Lung Disease*, 76: 17–19, 1994.

14. Shingvi, A. et al.: 'The prevalence of markers for hepatitis B and human immunodeficiency viruses, malarial parasites and microfilaria in blood donors in a large hospital in South India', *Journal of Tropical Medicine and Hygiene*, 93: 178–82, 1990.

15. Kumarasamy N. et al.: 'First report of Kaposi's sarcoma in an AIDS patient from Madras, India', *Indian Journal of Dermatology*, 41(1): 23–5, 1996.

followed by heart diseases, cancer (+23.56 per cent) and pulmonary diseases, including TB (+18.32 per cent). However, within this last category, the proportion of deaths caused by tuberculosis grew from 45.5 per cent in 1986 to 51.7 per cent in 1994. Thus, in 1994, tuberculosis accounted for more than half of the deaths caused by pulmonary diseases.

The increase in cancer and heart diseases seems to be 'normal' and reflects what has already been said about the epidemiological transition: more older people living longer and thus suffering from these types of diseases. But the growing proportion of tuberculosis as well as the increase of hepatitis could point to the HIV epidemic because of their dangerous link with it.

Different Patterns According to the Wards

Analysis of the dynamics of these causes of death in the period 1986–94 at the ward level reveals some particular trends (Figure 8). Each graph combines the proportion of deaths caused by a particular disease in 1986 and in 1994. Some graphs confirm the trends observed at the Brihan Mumbai scale:

• Heart diseases: Increase.
  Exceptions: wards A, B, D, E and G-North.
• Hepatitis: Increase.
  Exceptions: wards M-West, P-South and R-South.
• Diarrhoea: Decrease.
  Exceptions: wards B, D, E and G-South.

Other graphs concentrate the trends of the Mumbai scale in particular wards.

• Cancer: Increase (only in wards F-South, G-North, H-East, H-West, K-West, L, M-East, P-North, R-North, S and T).
• Other diseases: Increase (only in wards C, K-West, L, M-East, P-South and R-South).

Regarding the pulmonary diseases, the analysis is very interesting: the mortality caused by tuberculosis is increasing in all the

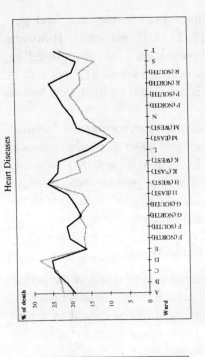

Cancer

% of death — 7, 6, 5, 4, 3, 2, 1, 0

Ward: A, B, C, D, E, F (NORTH), F (SOUTH), G (NORTH), G (SOUTH), H (EAST), H (WEST), K (EAST), K (WEST), L, M (EAST), M (WEST), N, P (NORTH), P (SOUTH), R (NORTH), R (SOUTH), S, T

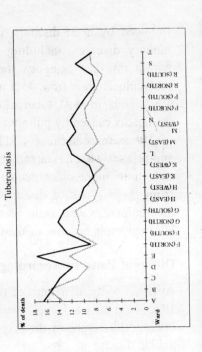

Heart Diseases

% of death — 30, 25, 20, 15, 10, 5, 0

Ward: A, B, C, D, E, F (NORTH), F (SOUTH), G (NORTH), G (SOUTH), H (EAST), H (WEST), K (EAST), K (WEST), L, M (EAST), M (WEST), N, P (NORTH), P (SOUTH), R (NORTH), R (SOUTH), S, T

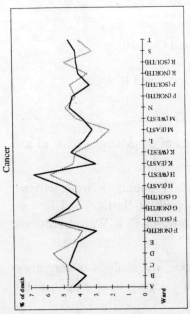

Pulmonary Diseases (excluding tuberculosis)

% of death — 10, 9, 8, 7, 6, 5, 4, 3, 2, 1, 0

Ward: A, B, C, D, E, F (NORTH), F (SOUTH), G (NORTH), G (SOUTH), H (EAST), H (WEST), K (EAST), K (WEST), L, M (EAST), M (WEST), N, P (NORTH), P (SOUTH), R (NORTH), R (SOUTH), S, T

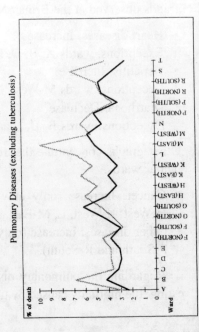

Tuberculosis

% of death — 18, 16, 14, 12, 10, 8, 6, 4, 2, 0

Ward: A, B, C, D, E, F (NORTH), F (SOUTH), G (NORTH), G (SOUTH), H (EAST), H (WEST), K (EAST), K (WEST), L, M (EAST), M (WEST), N, P (NORTH), P (SOUTH), R (NORTH), R (SOUTH), S, T

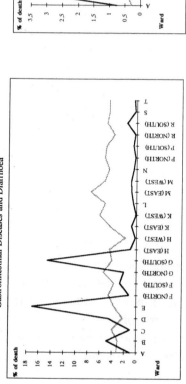

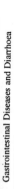

FIGURE 8: Evolution of mortality for seven important causes of death between 1986 and 1994 ward-wise in Brihan Mumbai.

.... Percentage of deaths caused by disease in 1986.
— Percentage of deaths caused by disease in 1994.

wards, except in wards B and K-East—where decreasing rates are observed—whereas the other pulmonary diseases reveal a decrease in all the wards, except in G-South, G-North and M-West.

Thus, the analyses at the ward scale reveals a dual pattern: an increase of 'degenerative' deaths (heart disease and cancer) as well as an increase in almost all Brihan Mumbai of tuberculosis.

Tuberculosis, Diarrhoea and Hepatitis: Indicators of the spread of HIV?

From this analysis, it seems to be useful to divide the causes of death into two groups. The first group includes 'HIV indicators' because they are well known for their link with HIV (tuberculosis, hepatitis and diarrhoea). Moreover, they present very high increases in almost all Brihan Mumbai wards over the period 1986–94. Diarrhoea is also included in this group because it is a well-known symptom of HIV infection and because very high increases are noted in some particular wards, which seem to be abnormal.

The second group covers the other studied diseases. This group includes 'non-HIV indicators'. Their links with HIV are not proved, except for some special types of tumours. They also present particular patterns at the ward scale: either an increase in most of the Mumbai wards (as in heart diseases), or an increase concentrated in some particular wards (as in cancer) or a general decrease (as in pulmonary diseases—excluding tuberculosis—and other diseases).

The analysis of changes in these groups between 1986 and 1994 reveals two facts (Figure 9): on the one hand, a concentration of the 'HIV indicators' in the central and southern parts of Brihan Mumbai, and on the other hand, a concentration of the 'non-HIV indicators' in the northern parts of the metropolis. In this area, only three wards reveal an increase of the two types of causes of death: wards M-East, H-West and R-South.

INDICATOR GROWTH BETWEEN 1986 AND 1994

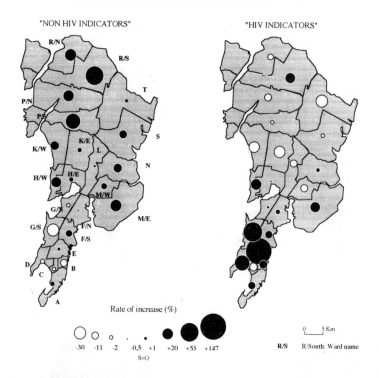

FIGURE 9: Indicator Growth between 1986 and 1994.

This trend is slightly confirmed by the maps in Figure 10 which present the percentage of the deaths per ward due to the 'HIV indicators' as well as that caused by 'non-HIV indicators' in 1986 and in 1994. Regarding the year 1986, calling these diseases 'HIV indicators' might be inappropriate, although the HIV epidemic had probably infected some people in India by then.

The maps reveal that the proportion of deaths caused by 'HIV indicators' was more important in 1994 in the southern part of Brihan Mumbai. In 1986, some wards had already a high proportion of deaths due to tuberculosis, hepatitis and diarrhoea (especially wards A, B, E and G-North). But, even in the latter, the proportion was higher in 1994. For instance, in ward E, the percentage was 16.23 per cent in 1986 and 37.37 per cent in 1994. In

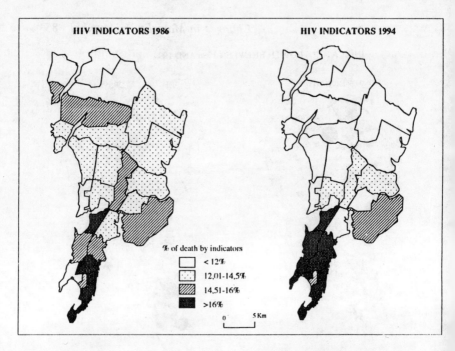

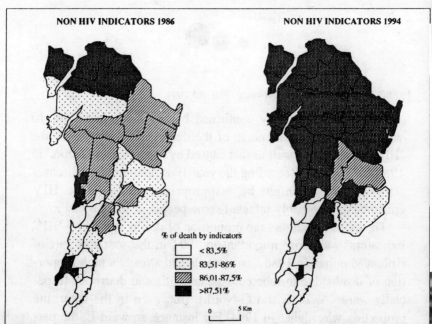

FIGURE 10: Percentage of deaths caused by HIV indicators and Non-HIV indicators in 1986 and 1994.

the other parts of Brihan Mumbai, the proportion was lower or at the same level (as in ward M-East) in 1994 than in 1986.

Regarding the 'non-HIV indicators', the proportion was higher in the northern parts of Brihan Mumbai. In these areas, wards R-North and R-South already had high proportions in 1986—88.92 and 87.98 per cent respectively; and 91.18 and 89.9 per cent respectively in 1994. In the central and southern wards of the metropolis, the 1986 proportion was higher than in 1994, except in three wards: C, F-South and F-North.

Finally, if we correlate all this information with the two groups observed earlier in this chapter: group 1, where 'abnormal mortality' was noted, and group 2, where the mortality and the population growth were linked, several patterns can be observed (Figure 11).

In the first group, there are two patterns. Five wards reveal a higher increase of 'HIV indicators' than 'non-HIV indicators' (1.1): wards E, D, H-West, F-South, and F-North. For instance, in ward E, a decrease of cancer, other diseases, pulmonary diseases (excluding tuberculosis) and a slight increase of heart diseases were observed, whereas hepatitis, diarrhoea and tuberculosis increased at alarming rates. The clear implication is of wards where HIV was widespread.

The second pattern (1.2) groups together wards in which the increase of 'non-HIV indicators' was lower than that of the 'HIV indicators'. Here, the proportion of deaths due to 'non-HIV indicators' was still high. Thus, the 'abnormal mortality' seems to be linked with an increase of cancer or/and heart diseases, or/and pulmonary diseases (except tuberculosis) or/and other diseases. In wards R-South and R-North, the HIV epidemic might have started to contaminate people because the HIV indicators were increasing.

In the second group also, two patterns were observed: on the one hand, wards with a decrease of 'HIV indicators' and an increase of 'non HIV-indicators' (2.1). The mortality was still due to heart disease, cancer, pulmonary and other diseases. On the

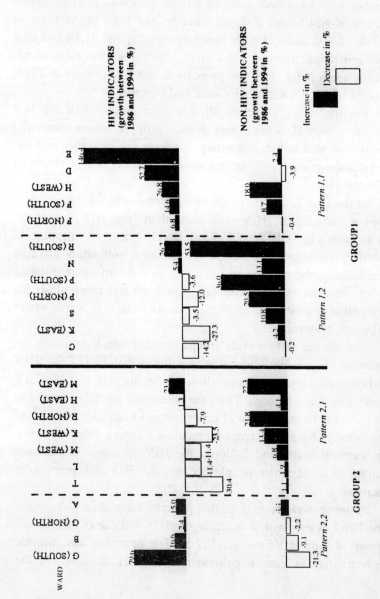

FIGURE 11: Matrix: 'HIV'/'Non-HIV' indicator growth.

other hand there were four wards (2.2) (G-South, B, G-North and A) in which the increase of tuberculosis, hepatitis and diarrhoea was higher than the 'non-HIV indicators'. However, these wards had presented a pattern of 'normal mortality', though tuberculosis, diarrhoea and hepatitis became main causes of death in 1994. That means that these diseases took the place of cancer, heart disease, pulmonary and other diseases, despite a mortality increase linked with the population growth.

Socioeconomic Status of the Populations

In Mumbai, the population settlement is linked with the different industrial periods of the metropolis. The poorest and the middle classes are concentrated in the centre and the east of the city whereas the high income groups have settled in the west, protected by the wind, from the industrial areas of the rest of the peninsula. Thus, according to the present study, the eastern and central wards seem to be more infected by HIV although the western wards, especially in the north, could also be infected.

Nevertheless, this level of analysis must hide disparities because within each ward, populations are very mixed together. For instance, in ward D, the villas and apartments of the highest income groups from Malabar and Cumbala Hills are side-by-side with the chawls of the low income groups.

Correlations

1. With HIV data (Figure 12)
This correlation matrix tries to analyse the statistical link between the HIV prevalence and the increase of the 'HIV indicators', both at the ward scale. The Bravais-Pearson coefficient (r) has been used to describe the hypothetical link between these two sets of data. The closer it is to -1 or 1, the higher is the correlation. In this case, r is equal to 0.89. That means roughly that in 89% of the wards, there is a relationship between the increase of tuberculosis, diarrhoea and hepatitis and the HIV prevalence. Notably,

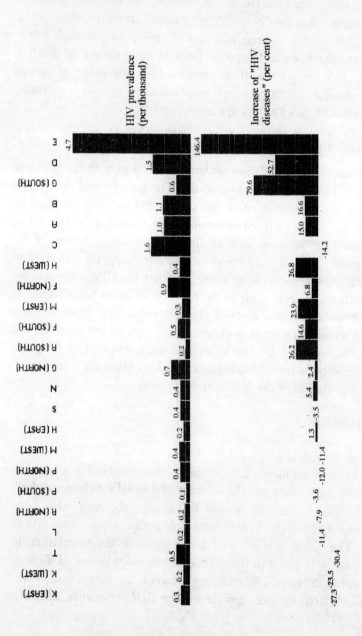

FIGURE 12: Matrix: HIV data and 'HIV diseases'.

wards E, D, B, A, C, F-North, G-North and G-South report particularly high HIV prevalences as well as high increases of 'HIV diseases'. Wards with negative 'HIV indicators' growth reveal low HIV prevalences even if HIV might have infected people.

These correlations indicate one important fact. Even if the data collection has not been completed in the northern parts of Brihan Mumbai, the analysis of the mortality partly proves that it was a good picture of the HIV spread in 1994.

2. With population density (Figure 13)
All these observed trends might be linked with high or low population density in each ward. This correlation matrix reveals three patterns. In the first one the correlation is high which means that in these wards the high number of HIV cases could be due to the high number of people per square kilometre. The third pattern reveals low HIV prevalences and low densities. Finally, the second pattern groups together wards where density does not seem to be linked with HIV prevalences. These areas had a high proportion of surveyed hospitals. Thus, from this analysis it can be concluded that the high HIV prevalences reported in central Mumbai could be the 'image' of high densities. Particular socio-economic context, location of red–light areas, and particular sexual practices, could also be reasons for these high reported numbers.

Conclusions

There are, however, shadows in this study. On the one hand, the causes of death by age group were not available for the period under study. These data are necessary to go further in the analysis. It can be expected, however, that the abnormal increase of deaths caused by tuberculosis, diarrhoea and hepatitis might have been linked to particular age groups.

On the other hand, this study reveals important facts and trends which might be used as keys for action; and the

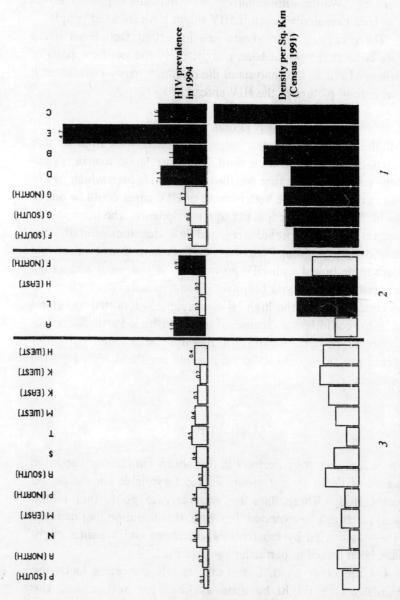

FIGURE 13: Matrix: HIV and population density.

methodological approach used is quite different from those used before.

According to this analysis, the HIV epidemic seemed to have infected especially the central parts of the city in 1994. The analysis of the mortality data suggests this; and in those wards, tuberculosis, diarrhoea and hepatitis—three important HIV markers—were increasing and becoming important causes of death. However, in some other parts of the city (wards M-East, R-South and N), high increases of these indicators were also noted. In the rest of the wards, cancer, heart disease, pulmonary and other diseases increased in 1994. Nevertheless, tuberculosis grew in all those wards. The increase of this disease might be the pointer to the HIV infection.

Finally, the highest mortality increases were reported for the young adults as well as teenagers. This trend is quite 'abnormal'. The HIV epidemic and its procession of opportunistic infections could have especially contaminated these age groups.

References

Banerjee U. et. al.; 'Cryptosporodial diarrhoea in a patient of AIDS in India', *CARC Calling*, Volume 5: 16, 1992.

Bharat, S.; *Facing the Challenge: household and community response to HIV/AIDS in Mumbai, India*, World Health Organisation, Geneva, 1996.

Mann J. et al.: *AIDS in the World*, Indian edition, Bombay, 1037pp, 1994.

Patel, S. and Thorner, A.: *Bombay: Metaphor For Modern India,* Oxford University Press, New Delhi, 288pp, 1996.

CHAPTER FOUR

Planning for the Socio-economic Impact of the Epidemic: The Costs of Being Ill

INDRANI GUPTA*

Introduction

It is increasingly being realised that the HIV/AIDS epidemic is likely to have a severe impact in many countries: on the economy, on the social development sectors, and on households and individuals. The direct loss in productivity, saving and, therefore, national income due to increased mortality and morbidity arising from the epidemic have been analysed by several researchers, (Kambou, Devarajan & Over, 1992; Over, 1992; Cuddington, 1993; Bloom & Mahal, 1997), and the evidence is mixed: while earlier studies found that the epidemic will lower the rate of growth of income in many countries, more recent analyses find this effect to be negligible.

Apart from these macro-studies, there have been attempts to measure the impact on the various sectors of the economy (see for example Giraud, 1992). The analysis of impact on African farming systems due to labour losses, by Barnett and Blaikie (1992) was one of the first of such studies, which was followed by other similar work for various countries. In Africa, evidence of impact on sectors like agriculture, education and transport are quite consistent in their implications: the HIV/AIDS epidemic is likely to adversely affect each of these sectors.

* The author would like to thank Mr Sathiamoorthy, without whose help this research would not have been possible. Mithilesh Kumar Jha provided expert research assistance.

Yet a third kind of study that has gained popularity with researchers in the recent past has been that of the impact of HIV/AIDS on individuals and households. In addition to the Barnett and Blaikie study of the Rakai district of Uganda mentioned above, a study jointly done by the World Bank and the University of Dar es Salaam (Ainsworth and Over, 1992) for the Kagera region of Tanzania added to the growing literature on the subject. Both looked at impact on, and the coping mechanisms of, households in the event of illness and death. Another set of similar studies for Asia was commissioned by the UNDP Regional Project on HIV/AIDS in New Delhi (UNDP 1992, OUP 1997), where interesting case studies from Thailand, Laos, the Philippines, India, Indonesia and Sri Lanka can be found.

In India, analyses of impact have been sporadic. Although a few researchers have attempted to study the impact on some sectors, the bulk of the work has been on impact at the individual and household levels. In addition to the UNDP work mentioned above, there are a few other micro-level studies (Bharat, 1996; Sathiamoorthy and Solomon, 1997). These studies find that the effect of the epidemic will be severe, especially arising from two important features: high treatment costs and social discrimination. Unfortunately, these initiatives have remained isolated efforts, and the findings have not translated into policy actions on impact alleviation, or even to large-scale discussions on the important issues.

It is often argued in India,[1] that the problem is not severe enough yet to make a significant impact, unlike in countries of Africa, where the epidemic has reached alarming proportions, and has become visible. Underlying this strand of argument is also the assumption that the likelihood of the infection spreading into the general population is quite small, so that not only the present but even the future is unlikely to see serious economy-wide repercussions. This assumption is in turn based on the belief that HIV is confined only to the so-called 'high-risk behaviour'

---

1. Also see Chapter 2 in the present volume (ed.).

groups like commercial sex workers, drug users and homo-
sexuals, who are seen as marginal both in the society and in the
economy.

The perception of a low-key epidemic, non-dramatic results of
macro- and sectoral studies, the inability of researchers to send
the right messages across and the inability of policy- and
decision-makers to interpret the messages of the micro-studies,
have resulted in an almost complete absence of policies relating
to impact alleviation. This omission has been a serious one, and
has resulted in a situation where hardly any attention is being
paid to the most immediate of all problems of the HIV/AIDS
epidemic: that large numbers of infected individuals and their
families are undergoing severe impact while they are still alive.
In addition to the focus on impact emanating from death, it is
important to focus on the impact during the period before death,
even before the onset of illnesses, but after the infection has been
acquired. This is not to say that there are no impacts after death,
but to highlight the fact that individuals and families need the
most assistance during these years preceding death if increasing
impoverishment is to be prevented.[2] Impact alleviation policies
would include both general policies in the health and development sectors, as well as specific policies targeted at the most
vulnerable groups. In this context, the lack of adequate health
insurance in India (see Ellis, Alam and Gupta 1997 for a review
of health insurance in India) throws light on a problem faced by
the population at large: most Indians incur high out-of-pocket
expenses for health care. While subsidising health care for all is
neither feasible, nor desirable, availability of health insurance

---

2. Conceptually, households facing prime-age adult illness and death can be
regarded in three groups: those whose resources are sufficient so that they can
absorb the impact—they cease moving forward economically, but do not slip
backwards; those whose resources were adequate before the impact, but who are
overwhelmed and now slip into poverty; and those without resources, the already
poor whose poverty deepens, or who collapse as viable households. It is the second
group who are most vulnerable within society, and who present the greatest
opportunity to *prevent* poverty.

will certainly go a long way in preventing impoverishment due to serious illnesses and diseases, including HIV and AIDS, and there is an urgent need to re-consider the possibility of privatising health insurance in India. In addition to formal insurance, other informal insurance schemes in the context of HIV/AIDS must necessarily rely on a unique feature of the epidemic: that the epidemic allows a number of healthy (and some not-so-healthy) years to the infected individual till death. This suggests that careful financial planning for the future can start early on, and can alleviate the hardships the individuals and their families must undergo from the time they start becoming progressively ill, till death.[3]

Why Focus on HIV/AIDS

It has often been argued that the focus on the HIV/AIDS epidemic is diverting attention from other health problems, many of them more serious. This argument may initially sound valid for a country like India where infectious and communicable diseases are still the major causes of morbidity and mortality. However, there are features unique to the HIV/AIDS epidemic that make it different from other illnesses in its socio-economic impact:

• *Extended and very high treatment costs.*
The treatment of opportunistic infections, as well as care during full-blown AIDS, are extremely expensive, as has been shown in many studies. This chapter presents fresh evidence from India on this aspect and indicates the consequent burden placed on individuals. It can be argued that treatment costs are also high for other diseases, especially if the economic status of the household is already low. This seems like a valid argument; however, the difference is that the treatment costs tend to escalate and do not

---

3. The implications of this for insurance purposes deserve a full study on their own (ed).

culminate in cure for HIV/AIDS, but have to be continued till death. This is true of some rare and not-so-rare diseases like cancer, but not the diseases that are the common causes of morbidity and mortality in India. A further reason why treatment costs tend to be high is that an individual goes through a series of different illnesses, due to opportunistic infections which need to be treated symptomatically, till death. This is a unique phenomenon of the epidemic.

- *The likelihood of multiple cases of HIV/AIDS within a household.*

The impact on the individual and household is further aggravated by the probability of household members transmitting HIV to each other. In India, figures indicate that the infection is now spreading primarily via the routes of husband-to-wife infections and from mother to child.

- *Death is preceded by a fairly long period of illness.*

While some other fatal diseases (like cancer) are also often preceded by long periods of illness, these are not that common in India yet, though admittedly on the increase. The most common diseases start and end quickly, in either recovery or death. The implications of living an increasingly unhealthy life for the infected individuals and their families are serious, as also the impact on the health system and on the community at large.

- *There is a long incubation period between infection and the appearance of the first opportunistic infection*

This means that the individual can lead a normal and healthy life for several years, yet with the knowledge that the future will bring illness and death. One serious implication of this is in the mental and emotional well-being of the affected persons, who would need all the help that they can get during this period. But a long period of relatively good health also means that the individual can take steps to prepare himself or herself and his/her family, financially or otherwise, for an expected future. Unlike other diseases which can strike any time, this is an aspect of the epidemic that should be realised and used in a productive fashion to alleviate impact.

- *HIV/AIDS primarily affects adults in their economically productive years*

Again, there is no single disease that targets overwhelmingly the population in the reproductive and economically productive age groups. The most direct demographic consequence of AIDS is an increase in prime-age adult mortality, which will have repercussions on economic growth, and increase dependency rates, with more elderly persons and orphans in the economy.

- *Unlike many other infections, HIV infection is largely the result of private decisions*

The other infectious and contagious diseases common in India like TB, diarrhoea etc. are largely due to circumstances outside the control of the individual, though admittedly preventive private measures could still be taken. But the most common mode of transmission of HIV—sex—is almost always completely a private decision, and prevention policies can at best be indicative, but cannot be enforced.

- *AIDS is fatal.*

The ultimate outcome of contracting HIV is death. Until a cure or a vaccine is found, the probability of death is one, barring a few exceptional cases worldwide of individuals leading healthy lives even many years after contracting the infection.

- *The disease is associated with high levels of discrimination and stigmatisation.*

All the points made above should be viewed against another unique feature of the HIV/AIDS epidemic, which is that, being infected with HIV is a stigma and results in severe discrimination. For a conservative society like India, this single point must be understood, not as an add-on to the other points, but as an integral part of the problem of severe impact: the presence of stigmatisation and discrimination aggravate impact and also make interventions that much more difficult.

The preceding discussion should not be taken to mean that the focus in India should shift to HIV and AIDS from other common communicable and infectious diseases; rather it is to emphasise that there may be dimensions to the epidemic that aggravate impact and that policies need to be carefully thought out taking account of these unique features.

How Severe is the Epidemic in India?

As has been noted in other places in this volume, figures for the actual prevalence or incidence of HIV in the country are lacking. To get an idea about the severity of the epidemic in India, projections are useful. Assuming prevention and control programmes had been effective in controlling the spread of the disease and there were no new infections after 1996; what would be the scenario in terms of deaths in the succeeding five years? A calculation was made using EPIMODEL, developed by Chin and Lwanga (WHO) to estimate cumulative AIDS and HIV cases. The model needs just two parameters: the year in which widespread infection started taking place and a recent estimate of numbers infected. The results are indicated in Table 1.[4]

If by December 1996 there were 3 million infected individuals, and no new infections occurred after 1996, the number of deaths each year is indicated in column 2 of the table. With infections continuing at the same rate beyond 1996, the number of deaths calculated by EPIMODEL are indicated in column 3. If the assumption is that there are about 6 million infections current-

---

4. The model assumes that after 11 years the progression rate of AIDS continues at the rate of 4% annually, so that about 20% of the initial cohort develop AIDS within 15 years, and about 90% within 20 years. Progression rates from AIDS to death are based on the following assumptions: cumulative survival is 50% during the year of diagnosis, 20% after 1 year, 5% after 2 years, and none after 3 years.

TABLE 1: Projections for AIDS deaths in India—after 1996

Year	AIDS deaths: 3 m infected		AIDS deaths: 6 m infected	
	No new infection	Infection continues	No new infection	Infection continues
1996	65,255	65,255	130,509	130,509
1997	103,493	103,493	206,987	206,987
1998	148,197	150,417	296,393	300,833
1999	188,842	204,470	377,683	408,941
2000	208,853	262,775	417,705	525,550
2001	212,987	321,786	425,973	643,572
Cumulative AIDS deaths by 2001	~ 1.0 m	1.17 m	1.98 m	2.34 million

ly, then the numbers of deaths each year without fresh infection and with new infections are indicated in columns 4 and 5 respectively.

Since estimates do indicate that cumulative infections would be at least 3 million if not more, an optimistic scenario would be the projections in the first two columns. However, since evidence also points to an increase in infection rates, column 3 is the likely path of mortality. It is clear that by the year 2001 the cumulative AIDS deaths in India would be at least 1 million, each year witnessing thousands of deaths. In fact, these numbers could be even higher if one assumes that the progression time from HIV to AIDS is shorter in India due to the general poor health and low immunity of the population at large. Also, unlike in the US, the use of life-prolonging drugs like AZT is virtually non-existent, implying that the average incubation period may be somewhat shorter.

It must be remembered that the net increase in deaths due to HIV or AIDS may be somewhat lower than these numbers imply: some of these deaths would have taken place in any case, captured in the average mortality rates of the population. However, since these are adults in the prime-age group, many of these deaths would not have taken place until many years later. This would be especially true if the infection is spreading into the relatively better-off sections of the society where premature morbidity and mortality may be lower. It is safe to say that a majority of these deaths would have been spread out over several decades rather than the next five years.

The above exercise was reported to drive home the point that India will witness the additional illnesses and deaths of thousands of individuals in the coming years; it is the impact of this event on individuals and their families that is the topic of the rest of the discussion in this chapter.

How Do We Study Impact?

The problem one immediately encounters in starting to analyse impact is that it is a subjective state of affairs. Individuals differ in their perceptions about what constitutes a difficult socio-economic situation, and there is no objective way of getting at this without getting into inter-personal comparisons. Secondly, even without HIV/AIDS, individuals may be socio-economically in a relatively worse off situation due to low income, poor education, and a host of other factors. Thus it might become difficult to differentiate between impact on individuals who are HIV positive and those who are not. Also, it is not clear whether making the distinction is even justified. Thirdly, there are several fronts on which individuals may need help: income, consumption, children's schooling, medical expenses, physical disability, emotional problems, and also to ward off discrimination. All these are aspects of the total impact, and it is important therefore to state clearly which aspect one is addressing.

As mentioned in the introduction, there have been three very interesting earlier studies, those by Sathiamoorthy and Solomon at the Y.R. Gaitonde Care Centre in Madras (1995); by Shalini Bharat, supported by the WHO Global Programme for AIDS, at the Tata Institute of Social Sciences in Bombay (1996); and a study commissioned by the UNDP Regional Project done by

Basu, Gupta and Krishna (1995). Since the objectives of these studies were very similar (though the methodologies were very different), a brief discussion of these is appropriate.

The study sponsored by the WHO Global Programme on AIDS was designed to study household and community responses to HIV/AIDS in predominantly lower income households in Greater Bombay. A sample of 39 households was selected and the interviews were done both at the level of the individuals who were positive as well as other members of the household. Indepth interviews were coupled with focus group discussions. The major findings of this study were that household responses were on the whole supportive and positive, but more so for male members than for female members. The needs of HIV positive individuals also differed along gender lines, males being more concerned about their own well-being while females were concerned about the family as a whole.

The survey by Sathiamoorthy and Solomon was conducted among people living with the virus, to determine the socio-economic consequence of being HIV positive. A total of 125 people living with the virus were interviewed on hardships they faced in supporting themselves and their families, and also on discrimination. The study found these persons suffered significant economic hardships, especially in treatment expenses, and had also to face widespread discrimination.

The Basu, Gupta and Krishna study was conducted in Delhi among young adults and probed the possible implications of HIV/AIDS in a hypothetical setting. In other words, respondents were asked to visualise the economic impact of a major illness and possible death. The use of major illness and death was made to serve as proxy for AIDS-related morbidity and mortality. The study used both quantitative and qualitative methods. Quantitatively, a survey was carried out to assess the potential impact of male adult morbidity. The analysis revealed that the economic status of a household was an important determinant of the subsequent severity of impact, i.e. poorer households were more vulnerable.[5]

Impact on the Individual

Keeping these findings in mind, a project was undertaken to study the impact of HIV/AIDS on the individual. The research was supported by the British Overseas Development Administration (re-named as the Department for International Development) and carried out by the Institute of Economic Growth, Delhi. A questionnaire was designed for HIV positive individuals to elicit the following information:

- the socio-economic profile of the individual affected;
- the direct economic impact on the individual measured mainly in terms of health costs in relation to their earnings and other consumption expenditure;
- the extent of these health costs borne by the individual, and costs borne by others;
- financial assistance received and its source;
- the extent of physical assistance and its source;
- discrimination at home, at the health facility, among neighbours, and friends;
- the likely source of infection, and current sexual practices.

Unlike other household surveys, it was not possible to make a scientifically designed survey due to the sparsity of cases of HIV positive individuals who openly admitted their status. Any individual even remotely uncomfortable about being interviewed, was excluded from the sample. The questionnaire was not a sensitive one; personal details about sexual life were not included,

---

5.   A very recent study on TB done by Holmes, Pathania and Almeida (1997) is very similar to these studies in the way it analyses the impact of TB on individuals. They find that repeated cycles of illness, wages lost and expenditure on treatment often lead to impoverishment.

barring a very brief section on source of infection. Instead, the survey sought to get information mostly about economic variables, with sections on physical assistance and discrimination. This paper is based on some selected findings of the research; for the full report see Gupta (1997).

Though this study shares some common features with the three previous ones, the present study is also dissimilar from these in many ways. The WHO study was done more from the point of view of studying household and community responses and was significantly enriched by in-depth interviews. The Sathiamoorthy and Solomon study was, on the other hand, very similar in spirit to the current one, but stopped short of a quantitative analysis. The Delhi study, while very interesting, was a hypothetical one. Apart from these minor differences, there are some basic differences between the present study and the previous ones.

Firstly, the objective of this study is to analyse the magnitude of impact, and not merely to indicate that impact exists. Secondly, a key feature in this study is an attempt to define impact in such a way as to enable the respondent's perception about his/her economic situation to be included in the analysis. The analysis then linked this subjective set of responses to an objective set of variables to estimate the magnitude and variations in impact, using a probit analysis.

Before summarising the results, an important caveat should be pointed out. Ideally, one should be analysing the impact of HIV and AIDS by including 'controls' in the sample, i.e. individuals who are not HIV positive. This would allow estimation of the relative burden of being HIV positive versus other adult illnesses. However, the survey was designed specifically to elicit information on all other (besides financial) aspects of hardships including illnesses and discrimination for those who are HIV positive. This limited the scope for a more general analysis, which is definitely recommended for further research on impact. However, the results of the analysis remain important and interesting, because, as the analysis below will indicate, it brings out the importance of targeting due to differential impact on the one hand, and the need to correct the deficiencies in the current system of policies and legislations in India which aggravate the plight of vulnerable households, on the other.

Socio-economic Characteristics of the Sample

A total of 167 individuals were interviewed from different states of India depending upon accessibility and availability of respondents. A majority of the respondents were from the South Indian states of Andhra Pradesh and Tamil Nadu.

The mean age of the sample population was 33 years, the youngest being 19 and the oldest 65. The majority (82 per cent) were males; 64 per cent of all the individuals were currently married, while 32 per cent were single. Of those currently married, divorced or widowed, 72 per cent had at least one child.

The education level of the sample population was very high. About 53 per cent of the respondents had at least a bachelor's degree.

Respondents were asked about their employment status: whether or not they had ever worked as an employee, whether they are working now, if they had ever owned a business, and if the earnings from either employment or business had been affected since they became HIV positive. It must be emphasised here that the purpose of the income and earnings section as well as the expenditure section was to arrive at only a rough estimate of these variables and not to probe in detail into their living standards. As is quite well-established by now, accuracy of income and expenditure aggregates can only be achieved by asking detailed questions, as is done in the well-known World Bank Living Standard Measurement Surveys (LSMS). For the present survey it was sufficient to be able to derive broad orders of magnitude on income and expenditure variables.

Most of the respondents were salaried employees and few owned or had ever owned a business. Of those who had ever worked, the majority reported that they were still working. The mean earnings of the sample were above the per capita earnings of the country, indicating, along with the educational characteristics, that these individuals were socio-economically quite advanced. A small percentage (8 per cent), of the sample reported that they had never worked. Of these more than half were males, and all of them said they were being supported by their parents.

Of the respondents, 36 per cent said they were supporting someone else or contributing to household expenditure before they became infected; thus the majority of individuals had only themselves to support.

The expenditure section asked about the various health and non-health related expenditures in detail. In Table 2 the means of various categories of expenditure are given. It should be kept in mind that the means have been calculated by including individuals who reported no expenditure because they live with their relatives.

The third column reports the share of each item in total non-health expenditure. The two most important items of expenditure reported were on food and on personal items, with rent being quite a significant share of the total. These patterns are as expected, and in fact the share of food is lower than what it would be if incomes were lower. Still, food and rent are essential expenditures, and so are utilities; this is important to bear in mind when analysing the effect of increased expenditure on health.

TABLE 2: Expenditure patterns

Expenditure category	Monthly expenditure (Rs)	% in total
Food	1,049	44
Personal*	495	25
Rent	962	21
Utilities	274	10
Total non-health expenditure	2,257	–

*This includes items like expenditure on clothes, shoes, and other personal items.

The brief background described above is a direct refutation of the claim that HIV has only spread into the so-called 'high-risk' groups; the socio-economic status of the 167 individuals is that of a group of relatively better-off individuals, with relatively high (compared to national averages) earnings, expenditure, and education, which is not generally associated with individuals in 'high-risk' occupations. While the sample is not a randomly selected one, the numbers are large enough to reject the hypothesis that the middle-class has been spared the spread of the infection. This finding is consistent with reports from the major cities of India.

The Health of Respondents

Illness and expenditure on illness play a major role in explaining the severity of the impact. It was therefore thought useful to discuss the health and health expenditures of respondents in some detail.

Length of Infection

Since the focus of the survey was the impact of HIV/AIDS on individuals, the health section asked in detail about the number and types of illnesses experienced by the respondent after he/she contracted the virus; any condition, including ordinary ones like headache or fever, were recorded.

Of the 167 individuals interviewed, 37 per cent reported at least one or more condition since contracting the virus; the remaining 63 per cent had not suffered from any illnesses at the time of the interviews. Thus a majority of the respondents were asymptomatic up to the time of the interviews, and no one in the sample had full-blown AIDS.

Though evidence varies on the average time between contracting the infection and the appearance of the first illness, these data gave an opportunity to test this independently. Before presenting these results however, it is necessary to bring another very important variable into the analysis: namely, the time since the individual was infected.

The survey asked all the respondents whether or not they knew when they became infected. The data revealed the disconcerting result that most individuals, about 85 per cent, did not know when they became infected. The average number of months since the infection for the sub-sample of those who knew when they were infected was about 40, i.e. about 3 years and 4 months. Those who did not know when they became infected were asked how long they had known about their infection. The average for this sub-sample was 26 months, i.e. 2 years and 2 months, and, as expected, the latter period is less than the former.

Since the variable on length of infection is the key to the analysis, a proxy variable had to be constructed for those who did not know the actual length of time they had been infected. For this group the time since they have known has been taken as the proxy variable since there was no other good variable that could be used, though this would undoubtedly bias the average downwards. Having stated this caveat, the rest of the analysis will use the label 'incubation period' for this constructed variable.

The average incubation period in the sample was about three years for those who stated at least one illness; for those who did not yet show any illness, this period was two years, indicating that for this sub-sample, a sizeable number might already have started showing illnesses at the time of writing this paper, almost a year after the initial survey. These averages may be slightly lower because of the way the incubation period variable was constructed.

Turning now to the kind of illness reported, up to four distinct conditions were reported, with the majority reporting only one or two distinct conditions. As mentioned before, about 63 per cent of the respondents reported no illness or condition, and 37 per cent reported one or more conditions. Thus this sample comprises a relatively 'new' sample in terms of the progress of the infection. This also implies that impact in a more 'mature' sample can always be expected to be more than what one finds in this group; i.e. the same individuals will display greater adverse impact with the passage of time.

Types of Illnesses

The common first condition reported was TB. Among the other important clinical conditions reported were herpes zoster, herpes simplex and candidiasis. These findings are entirely consistent with other reports of common opportunistic infections found in India. Most respondents mentioned more general illnesses, which could be either because the doctors did not diagnose the clinical conditions, or did not convey the names to the respondents. It is also possible that the respondents did not remember the exact names. It is interesting to note that many individuals said they suffered from headaches, fatigue or fever. These could be the precursors to more serious conditions. Diarrhoea was another very common condition mentioned along with other stomach problems.

Health Expenditure

Health expenditure was broken down into five broad heads: consultations, diagnostics, in-patient care, medicines, and transport costs of health care (Table 3). The last category, an often omitted one, was deliberately included since several trips to the doctor can also be expensive if the health facility is not very close.

TABLE 3: Health expenditure (all conditions)

Type	Mean in Rs	Share in total
Consultations	291	20%
Diagnostics	559	18%
In-patient care*	–	–
Medicines	3025	54%
Transport	142	7%

*Only two people reported in-patient costs, thus the mean has not been reported here.

The information was collected from each individual for each illness. Five individuals reported some expenditure incurred though he/she did not report any specific illness. It is most probably true that the knowledge of infection prompted visits to a doctor which resulted in some expenditure. On the other hand there were four individuals who were sick but did not incur any expenditure on health care. The latter could be an interviewer error, or a genuine lack of demand for health care for these individuals. However, if it is the latter, the number is not large enough to vitiate the conclusion that individuals *do* seek medical care for their illnesses.

As Table 3 indicates, 54 per cent of the expenditure was on medicines, the next in importance head of expenditure being consultations and diagnostics respectively. Very few respondents reported in-patient expenditure, but this could be due to the sample being of relatively recent infections. This would definitely be higher in a sample with more individuals in more advanced stages of infection. Finally, transport costs were 7 per cent of total health expenditure, which is not an insignificant amount.

Another notable feature is the fact that only three (among all those who reported health expenditure) said they had some source of funds besides their own for health expenditure. Most individuals said they spent out of their own pockets for health care costs. The varying abilities of individuals to adopt risk-sharing mechanisms is an important point to keep in mind while targeting vulnerable populations.

The Socio-economic Impact of HIV

As discussed above, there are several ways of looking at 'impact'. Here we contend that the most severe and immediate economic impact emanates from treatment costs incurred by the individual. High treatment expenses will imply lower expenditure on other essentials, like food. In case the individual is forced to leave his/her job, the impact will be even more severe.

Treatment costs

Unlike other household surveys where detailed questions are asked about chronic and acute illnesses during a reference period, this survey was very different in that it asked about every episode of illness since the individual acquired HIV. Thus the expenditure need not be during one year and therefore cannot be compared directly to annual income and expenditure. However, here an attempt is made to gauge the cost of illness in comparison with income, as explained below.

There are several ways of looking at the impact of health expenditure in comparison with income on individuals. But let us suppose that individuals suffer from only one illness in one year, so that the expenditure reported by them can be taken as the annual expenditure. The average health expenditure of the group (over all illnesses) was Rs 4,481. The annual income of this group was Rs 37,968. This means that about 11 per cent of annual income of the group was spent on health. This is obviously an underestimate since individuals in the sample have already reported up to four distinct episodes or illnesses. Even so, 11 per cent is not a small fraction of income to spend on illness.

Another way of looking at the magnitude of health expenditure is to arrive at an average annual figure of health cost to the individual. The mean number of days of illness in the sample was 193 for those who reported any expenditure. Thus the mean health expenditure divided by the number of days an individual has been sick will give an average daily expenditure, which can be multiplied by 365 to arrive at an annual measure of expenditure on health. This is definitely a hypothetical example, because health expenditure tends to be lumpy, and not spread out so smoothly. But this way the calculations reveal that about 22 per cent of annual income was spent on health.

A third method is to look at the number of illness episodes. The sample indicated up to four illness episodes. Since there are fewer individuals reporting three and four episodes, the averages are not very robust. In these calculations, instead of taking the actual means of expenditure for each episode, we assume that every time an illness strikes, the individual spends an amount equal to the amount spent on the first episode. Thus while having only one illness in a year means spending 8 per cent of the person's income, having two, three and four illnesses would imply spending 18, 27 and 35 per cent respectively of income on treatment, under the assumption that all the illnesses occur during the same year. This assumption will be less valid for those individuals who are yet relatively healthy, but will definitely be valid the greater the time since infection, because the opportunistic infections will strike more frequently in individuals who have acquired the infection earlier. Also, even for those who have more than one infection or illness each year, these numbers are likely to be underestimates, since the severity of illness increases as the infection progresses, and treatment becomes more expensive. Thus annual expenditure on health may end up being higher than individual income for more advanced cases of infection.

In sum, health expenditure will increasingly strain the economic status of the individuals as time progresses, and illnesses start manifesting themselves. The longer the time since infection, the higher will be the economic impact emanating from treatment costs alone, and individuals will have to devote a larger share of income to health and less to other essential items of consumption. Individuals may need to prepare themselves ahead of time by setting aside a significant part of their income, depending on the income and the anticipated health costs. Planning should start from the day the individual knows that he/she is HIV positive; and estimating the number of years since the infection would allow the individual to estimate the number of healthy as well as unhealthy years to come. This should be the planning horizon which will allow financial planning and spread out the impact rendering the financial burden more bearable.

There are some obvious points that can be raised around the preceding discussion. Individuals often get assistance from various sources, and in fact many live with their families and close relatives as in this sample. This means that the financial burden of treatment costs can be shared. While this is true, the point here is that it is untenable to sustain this kind of expenditure for long, especially during the relatively unhealthy periods when the person may not be as productive and when treatment costs will be very high. It is certainly true that the impact will be less on one person if others share the cost; but it is unlikely that such high expenditure can be sustained by even the very close relatives of the individual. It is also important to remember that many individuals themselves support others in the family. Table 4 gives the percentage of respondents who received assistance and the percentage who said they supported anyone besides themselves with their own income.

As the table shows, only 23 per cent said they were receiving any financial assistance from outside; 36 per cent said they were supporting someone else besides themselves prior to becoming infected; and 77 per cent said they were still able to continue support to that person. The kinds of support most affected were contributions to household expenditure like food, and support to parents or one's spouse. This also implies that most individuals were supporting themselves with their own income. The other point to note is that with increasing costs of treatment as frequency of illness increases, more and more individuals will be unable to support anyone else with their income. This will impose economic hardships on those who are now supported by the infected individuals. Whichever way one looks at it, high treatment costs will impose a burden: on the individual, on those who support him/her, and on those whom the individual supports financially.

TABLE 4: Financial assistance received & lent

% receiving assistance currently	23
% supporting others prior to infection	36
% able to continue support	77

Factors Affecting Economic Impact

As mentioned before, the fundamental problem one encounters in analysing impact is to define a variable that will capture individual 'impact'. In this analysis we looked at three variables to construct a binary variable for economic impact.

Individuals were asked three questions:

- Whether or not they were receiving any assistance and, if they were, whether they needed more assistance.
- Those who said they were not currently receiving any assistance were asked whether they would like to receive assistance.
- Individuals were also asked whether they were supporting anyone prior to their infection, and whether they were unable to continue the support.

If the answer to any one of these variables was 'yes', i.e. individuals needed support, or needed more support or if they were having difficulty in continuing support to others, the variable for impact would be 1, else it would be zero. Thus the impact variable in this analysis is a binary variable, taking on just two values, 0 or 1; 1 implying that there is financial impact, and 0 implying that there is no impact. The useful feature of this variable is that it takes into account the individual's perception about his/her economic status, but at the same time links up this seemingly subjective variable to objective and measurable variables on socio-demographic and health characteristics, so that it turns out that the perceptions are not that subjective after all.

This variable bypasses another problem: it allows individuals who are not HIV positive to also state whether or not they are experiencing an impact, whether from other illness, or any other economic problems. Thus everyone in the sample is allowed to state whether they are feeling an economic impact.

Suppose that the lack of economic hardship or impact yields utility to each individual. Thus for individual i the benefit of no economic impact is y^*. This benefit is a function of several variables, denoted by X_i. Thus,

$$y_i^* = \beta'X_i + \varepsilon_i \qquad \ldots (1)$$

However, this net benefit y_i^* cannot be directly observed; i.e. the net benefit of not undergoing economic impact cannot be observed from the data. However, the variable that can be observed is the one discussed above, whether or not an individual perceives that he/she is undergoing economic hardship. In other words, we only observe whether or not there is impact. Let y be the variable that takes the values of either 0 or 1, 0 denoting impact, and 1 denoting no impact;[6] in other words, positive net benefits signify that there is no impact on the individual. Therefore,

$$y_i = 1 \text{ if } y_i^* > 0 \text{ and } y_i = 0 \text{ if } y_i^* \leq 0 \qquad \ldots (2)$$

Following from equation (2) we can write the probability of positive net benefits or the probability of no impact in the following way:

$$
\begin{aligned}
\text{Prob } [y_i^* > 0] &= \text{Prob } [y_i = 1] \\
&= \text{Prob } [\beta'X_i + \varepsilon_i > 0] \\
&= \text{Prob } [\varepsilon_i > -\beta'X_i] \\
&= 1 - F(-\beta'X_i) \qquad \ldots (3)
\end{aligned}
$$

F is the standard normal cumulative distribution function of the form shown in equation (4), which is distributed with a mean zero and a variance equal to 1. Thus,

---

6. Though it is easier to think of impact happening as y being equal to 1, we define $y = 0$ to imply that there is impact and $y = 1$ to imply the positive outcome of no impact, to be consistent with the notations and literature on probit. It should be noted that it does not matter which outcome is defined as zero, since the coefficients would be the same with the opposite sign.

$$F(-\beta'X_i) = \int_{-\infty}^{-\beta'X_i} 1/(2\pi)^{\frac{1}{2}} \exp(-t^2/2) \, dt \qquad \dots (4)$$

The log likelihood function can be written as in equation (5) below:

$$\ln L = \prod_{y_i=0} F(-\beta'X_i) \prod_{y_i=0} F[1 - F(-\beta'X_i)] \qquad \dots (5)$$

Since equation (5) is highly non-linear, maximising this requires an iterative solution to estimate the coefficients.

The alternative specifications tested whether or not these variables were significant in explaining impact: age, sex, education, marital status, presence of children, length of infection, whether or not ill, days of sickness, and income. A maximum likelihood probit using the Newton-Raphson maximising routine was used to estimate these alternative models. In Table 5 results from five alternative specifications tested are presented. Since it is easier to think of $y=1$ as there being impact and $y=0$ as no impact, the estimations were based on this binary classification. It should be noted that due to symmetry, the results do not change except for the signs of the coefficients.

In the columns marked 1–5, the coefficients from the probit model are reported along with the t-statistics (at 5 per cent significance level) in brackets. It needs to be mentioned here, that the predicted probability estimated by the model was very close to the actual percentage of 'successes', indicating a good fit.

The basic difference among the five specifications is in the use of the education variables and the number of days of sickness variables. All the models yield almost identical results on the different variables. Age, gender, presence of children, whether or not the individual is ill, and income are all significant.

Age is negatively related to economic impact, implying that older individuals in the sample tended to be somewhat less affected than younger individuals. This reflects the fact that older

TABLE 5: Probit results on economic impact
Dependent variable $y = 1$ (Impact), $y = 0$ (No impact)

Variables	1	2	3	4	5
Constant	1.1	1.2	1.1	1.0	1.1
	(1.9)	(2.1)	(1.7)	(1.6)	(1.7)
Age	−.04	−.04	−.04	−0.4	−0.4
	(−2.0)	(−2.2)	(−2.2)	(−1.9)	(−2.2)
Sex = 1 if female	−.91	−.87	−.87	−.92	−.87
	(−3.0)	(−2.9)	(−2.9)	(−3.0)	(−2.9)
Children, yes/no	.97	.97	1.0	.97	.98
	(3.3)	(3.3)	(3.4)	(3.3)	(3.3)
Illness, yes/no	1.2	1.0	1.0	1.2	1.0
	(4.3)	(4.3)	(4.3)	(4.3)	(4.3)
Income	−.0001	−.0001	−.0001	−.0001	−.0001
	(−2.8)	(−2.7)	(−2.7)	(−2.8)	(−2.6)
Secondary education	–	–	–	.003	.06
				(.008)	(.16)
College education	–	–	–	−.08	.09
				(.26)	(.30)
Secondary & above	–	–	.16	–	–
			(.63)		
Number of days sick	−.0007	–	–	−.0008	–
	(−1.1)			(−1.1)	
Days since positive	−.008	.008	.008	.008	.008
	(1.4)	(1.4)	(1.3)	(1.4)	(1.4)

individuals probably have more income, more savings or both, by virtue of their being longer in the labour market. Typically, younger persons care less about financial planning than older people. Women were less affected than males in the sample, which could be due to the fact that men are more often the head of the household and spend on themselves and others, whereas women, especially if married (the sample comprised mostly married women), were financially somewhat more secure than men. Those with at least one child felt greater impact than those without one.

Income was again significantly negatively related to impact, i.e. the higher the income the lower will be the impact, as expected. Education was not significant in any equation, whether used as one variable (higher secondary or more), or used as dummies for secondary and college education separately, implying that more highly educated individuals were not significantly differently affected than those without much education. Again, the number of days since the individual has been positive was not significant in explaining impact, nor were the number of days an individual has been sick. This last result mentioned may seem contradictory at first, but could be due to the fact that expenditure per illness episode varied widely among individuals, depending on the region, and the kind of facility visited. Thus merely the number of days a person has been sick may not explain fully the variation in health expenditure.

Finally, whether or not the individual was ill had a very significant and positive effect on economic impact. Thus while individuals who were younger, male, had children and were relatively poorer, were feeling the need for assistance, those who were additionally also ill, were experiencing significantly higher impact.

This last result may seem obvious at first, but is actually more revealing than casual observation would suggest. Individuals in the sample were either healthy or unhealthy. The subjective feeling of impact (which could affect both healthy and unhealthy individuals) turned out to be not-so-subjective after all, since those who were ill experienced a greater probability of impact. These results also imply that individuals are not very good at coping with the event of illness. Further, it is also the case that economically vulnerable individuals tend to become even more vulnerable with the start of illness. The variable that explains this is the expenditure on health. This was not used as an explanatory variable because income has already been used on the right hand side. Also, whether or not the individual was ill was sufficient information for this purpose.

Since the underlying distribution is a normal distribution, interpretation of probit coefficients is not straightforward. For example, the coefficient on age in specification 5 is −.04; this is to be interpreted as saying that each one-unit increase in age leads to increasing the probit index by −.04 standard deviations. Since this is not intuitively clear, a transformation of the results in terms of changes in probability is more useful.

In Table 6, the change in probability for an infinitesimal change in the explanatory variables has been reported for just one specification (specification 5) to get a feel for the results. For the dummy variables among the explanatory variables, the numbers should be interpreted as the difference in predicted probability due to a change in the dummy variable from 0 to 1.

One of the most significant findings of the analysis is that the difference in predicted probability of impact if the individual is ill and if he/she is not ill is 0.37, which is quite high; i.e. economic impact is likely to be 37 per cent higher among those who are ill. It is also interesting to note that women experienced a 34 per cent lower probability of impact, which may be indicative of the fact that married women have somewhat higher financial security than unmarried younger males. Having a child increased the

Table 6: Change in probability

Variables	dF/dX
Age	−.02
Sex = 1 if female	−.34
Children, yes/no	.36
Illness, yes/no	.37
Income	−.00004
Secondary education	.022
College education	.037
Days since positive	.003
Observed P^*	.59
Predicted $P^\dagger$	.61

*P gives the mean probability of observing economic impact in the data.
$\dagger$The predicted probability is calculated at the mean of the independent variables, and dF/dX is calculated using the predicted probability.

probability by 36 per cent. However, a small change in income will change the predicted probability of impact by only a very small number, −.00004.

These results are interesting because they place impact in the proper policy perspective. HIV positive individuals will experience a drastic change in the magnitude of impact once they start falling sick. The need to plan will be greatest for those who are already in a somewhat vulnerable socio-economic status, who have children, or who are younger. These results imply that targeting the most vulnerable individuals to plan for impact alleviation would be the most cost-effective strategy.

Conclusions

This chapter has looked at a group of individuals who were HIV positive, and presented an analysis of the economic impact as it affected them. 'Impact' was analysed in two different ways: treatment costs in relation to income, and a probit analysis of factors affecting impact. The economic impact was defined in a unique fashion that allowed subjective statements of this impact to be verified using an objective method of analysis.

Treatment costs were found to be very high relative to income; between 10 and 30 per cent of the annual income of an individual may be spent on treatment of illnesses alone. The highest expenditure on health was incurred on medicines. Economic 'impact' was defined, based on perceptions of individuals as to whether or not they needed any or more assistance and whether they were able to continue support to others. An analysis of factors affecting the probability of impact revealed that younger individuals, males, individuals with lower income, those with at least one child, and those with at least one illness were more vulnerable to impact. The occurrence of at least one illness increased the probability of impact by 37 per cent. Males had a 34 per cent higher probability of impact than females, and those with at least one child had a 36 per cent higher probability of impact.

This evidence of impact has very significant policy implications. The high treatment costs are untenable for any individual, and especially for those without an adequate source of income or saving. One aspect of the analysis is that individuals experience severe hardship once the illnesses start, but have some time to plan for that eventuality, especially since there is no uncertainty about whether or not it will occur, only about when it will occur. The analysis indicates that targeting may be required after a careful study of the most vulnerable groups, and illness itself may be a criterion for targeting. Since resources would be limited, proper targeting would ensure cost-effective use of scarce resources.

Currently large sums of money are being spent on control and prevention programmes by the government, donor organisations, and NGOs, and almost nothing on impact alleviation. Health insurance in its current form is virtually non-existent in India and will certainly not cover HIV or AIDS in the near future. At the time of writing this paper, privatising health insurance is being discussed, but even if it takes place soon, it is unlikely that the many exclusion clauses that disallow coverage for HIV positive individuals all over the world are not going to be used here also. Highly specialised insurance schemes like those started recently by some companies in the USA will not serve the purpose in India because most people will not be able to afford them.

Under the circumstances, there is an urgent need to devote more resources, financial and otherwise, to both developing policies to ease hardship, and to actually implementing these policies. Innovative savings plans, including medical savings plans, income-generating programmes, need-based subsidised health care, as well as a re-consideration of the privatisation possibility in health insurance may be some of the options planners need to look at. In addition, policies in the health sector that make the health care system transparent and accessible[7], will ease the hardships individuals and families undergo while searching for

---

7.   The survey found very high levels of discrimination at medical facilities.

the appropriate medical facilities and personnel. In fact, part of the costs incurred takes place right after diagnosis, when individuals are unsure where to go for treatment and diagnosis.[8] One key to such planning, however, is the need to take the individuals affected by the epidemic into confidence and work with them to help them plan for an easier future, howsoever limited that future might be.

References

Ainsworth, Martha and Mead Over: 'Measuring the Impact of Fatal Adult Illness in Sub-Saharan Africa: An Annotated Questionnaire'. L SMS Working Paper No. 90, World Bank, 1992.

Barnett, Tony and Piers Blaikie: *AIDS in Africa : Its Present and Future Impact.* London: The Guilford Press, 1992.

Basu, Alaka M., Devendra B. Gupta & Geetanjali Krishna: 'The Household Impact of Adult Morbidity and Mortality: Some Implications of the Potential Epidemic of AIDS in India', in David Bloom and Peter Godwin, eds, *The Economics of HIV/AIDS*, Oxford University Press, Delhi, 1997.

Bharat, Shalini: *Household and Community Responses to HIV/AIDS*, WHO, Geneva, 1996.

Bloom, David E. and Ajay S. Mahal: 'The AIDS Epidemic and Economic Policy Analysis', in David Bloom and Peter Godwin, eds, *The Economics of HIV/AIDS*, Oxford University Press, Delhi, 1997.

Chin, James and Steve Lwanga: EPIMODEL, WHO, Geneva, 1991.

Cuddington, John T.: 'Modelling the Macroeconomic Effects of AIDS with an Application to Tanzania', *World Bank Economic Review* 7(2): 173–89, 1993.

Ellis, Randall, Moneer Alam and Indrani Gupta: *Health Insurance in India: Prognosis and Prospects*, Institute of Economic Growth, Delhi, 1997.

Giraud, Patrick: 'Economic Impact of HIV/AIDS on the Transport Sector: Development of an Assessment Methodology and Applying it to Thailand's Transport Sector', in David E. Bloom and Joyce V. Lyons, eds., *Economic Implications of AIDS in Asia*, UNDP, Delhi, 1992.

Gupta, Indrani: *Socio-economic Impact of HIV/AIDS an Individuals in India*, Department for International Development, British High Commission, New Delhi, 1997.

---

8. It should be noted that many of these policies will also help those who suffer from non-HIV-related illnesses.

Holmes C., Vikram Pathania & Joel Almeida: *The Impact of Tuberculosis on Individuals and Households in India*, WHO, Geneva, 1997.

Kambou, Gerard, S. Devarajan & Mead Over: 'The Economic Impact of AIDS in an African Country: Simulations with a General Equilibrium Model of Cameroon', *Journal of African Economics*, 1(1):109–30, 1992.

Over, Mead: 'The Macroeconomic Impact of AIDS in Sub-Saharan Africa', Technical Working Paper No. 3, World Bank, Africa Technical Department, Population, Health and Nutrition Division, Washington D.C., 1992

Sathiamoorthy, K. and Suniti Solomon: 'Socio-economic Realities of Living with HIV', in Peter Godwin ed., *Socio-Economic Implications of the Epidemic*, UNDP, New Delhi, 1997.

* * *

Discussion: The Personal Face of the Epidemic

PG: How do you find Indrani's work: showing this dramatic impact of illness?

S: Oh, she is right. In my own preliminary survey of costs with 47 people in Madras city, 14 women and 33 men, I found that treatment costs were 56 per cent of household expenditure—that is more than half of what the household was spending on survival. These costs were *not* primarily for hospitalisation or medical attention, but for buying medicines; with diagnostics and laboratory tests, and transportation accounting for the rest. Of their 'treatment costs', 59 per cent were for drugs, 33 per cent for laboratory tests and medical care, and the rest mainly for transportation. I can tell you, it is the spending on medicines that swamps everything.

PG: You had said something once to me about the problem of expenses even before illness. What were you referring to?

S: One of the most important effects of HIV/AIDS here in India starts right from the diagnosis. From my own personal experience and observation of others, people with HIV frantically start to search for treatment, for a cure, right from their day of diagnosis. Consequently they exhaust all their resources. Because of this, households experience some impact even before, or without any illness or death among their own members.

PG: Yes, I know that Indrani is aware of that, as we have discussed it. But I think she was trying to pinpoint the very specific, unavoidable economic crisis that being ill produces.

S: The impact, is, of course, more acute once the household is itself experiencing illness of one or more of its members. Most often, the ill person is a working adult; so what you might call the 'productivity' has been lost and other family members are forced to take up employment in addition to the burden of taking care of the sick member of the family. As is often the case, I have seen situations where the various household members are forced to dispose of their savings, investments, fixed deposits, etc to meet the care costs. This, in four instances I have personally come across, leaves the family without the means to support itself.

PG: One nice thing in Indrani's chapter is her consideration of more than simply economics; that impact has other dimensions.

S: The psychic costs of losing a parent or spouse are enormous. And it has severe economic implications also, in the deteriorating ability of the other family members to cope. But I have only, so far, come across one incident where the traditional coping mechanisms have broken down completely. This could be because HIV was very severe in that house. Three of the five members in that house, down in the south of Tamil Nadu, had died as a result of HIV infection, leaving a 3-year-old and a 7-year-old with their uncle, who is 57 years old.

PG: 'Positive Life' identifies the 'impact' of HIV as much greater than simply economic. One of the coordinators of 'Positive Life' describes some of the experiences they had in making a film:

'While making the film *Zindage Umeed Ke Saya Mein* based on the true story of a person living with HIV, we began to understand some of the many problems faced by people living with the virus. Some of these included:

- few or no support systems;
- inadequate and often hostile medical services;
- feelings of isolation which seemed to kill self-esteem and dignity;
- a fear of ostracism and exposure;
- lack of empowering information about life after HIV;
- lack of true negotiating power;
- use as figureheads by organisations working in HIV;
- creation of dependency;
- financial uncertainty.

We need to create an enabling environment for care, acceptance and inclusion of people living with HIV/AIDS and those directly affected in order that it enhances their quality of life.'

CHAPTER FIVE

Morbidity and Mortality Patterns in Hospitals: Monitoring the Impact of the Epidemic

S.C. CHAWLA, I. KOITHRA AND PETER GODWIN

Introduction

In 1996, an Epidemiological Round Table on HIV in India[1] concluded: 'Many international experts hold the view that India is now the epicentre of the global HIV pandemic. This may be so, but equally these predictions seem based on incomplete epidemiological information.... However, many scientists in India feel that the basis for the computation [is] faulty and grossly overestimates the quantum of the infection. Either school of thought may be right and the true prevalence may lie anywhere between the two estimates or even below or above them.' A recent evaluation of one major donor's regional HIV programme in recognition of this situation, recommended:[2] 'Of paramount urgency is the collection and analysis of data in the region, to inform decisions about prioritisation, and to determine the cost-effectiveness and cost benefit of initiatives and activities. [We] should collaborate very closely with other players... to ensure that this is done. Data need to be collected specifically in these areas:

---

1. Round Table on HIV/AIDS surveillance in India; August 11–13, 1996, organised by Network for Child Development with the help of AHEAD, supported by FHI/AIDSCAP and the USAID and co-sponsored by UNAIDS.

2. *Evaluation of the USAID Asia & Near EAst Bureau Regional HIV Program,* Health Technical Services, Washington, Mimeo, 1997.

- Social and behavioural sciences, particularly related to sexual behaviour, mortality patterns, economic aspects of adult mortality, and migration.
- Surveillance (both sentinel and point) of seroprevalence.
- Cost-benefit and cost-effectiveness of alternative approaches.
- Impact assessments in various sectors, particularly health, industry, insurance, and education.'

The issues raised by these two comments are vast, and will require the combined resources of many players. for several years if they are to be fully addressed.[3] Meanwhile, however, a number of relatively small-scale, yet critical steps can be taken, to make a significant contribution towards India's response to the epidemic. Particularly, there is some urgency in identification of the likely scope and scale of the impact of the significant increases in adult morbidity and mortality that the large number of HIV infections in the country will have,[4] specifically on provision of health services. A study of this problem in Kenya[5] found evidence of what the authors call 'rationing' of care. '... at the expense of HIV negative patients who were crowded out and displaced by HIV positive patients, and also experienced worse outcomes...' The authors asked: 'What will happen as the epidemic of HIV/AIDS illness (as opposed to infection) continues to grow? What can be done to cope with an unmeetable demand for health care that will be generated; and that will occur on top of the existing burden of ill-health that has not diminished in any way as the HIV epidemic has evolved? This is the real challenge.'

Information is required in a number of areas, much of which already exists, and needs only to be systematically collated and

3. Barney Cohen & James Trussel, eds, *Preventing and Mitigating AIDS in Sub-Saharan Africa; Research and Data Priorities for the Social and Behavioural Sciences.* National Academy Press, Washington DC, 1996.

4. P. Godwin ed: *Socio-economic implications of the Epidemic',* UNDP, 1997.

5. Katherine Floyd & Charles Gilks, 'Impact of, and response to, the HIV epidemic at Kenyatta National Hospital, Nairobi, Kenya, *Liverpool School of Tropical Medicine, Report 1*, April, 1996.

analysed. Other data may need to be specifically collected and analytical models developed.[6] For example, morbidity and mortality data from hospitals or health centres can be monitored for signs of changes in pattern that would indicate increases in adult morbidity and mortality arising from the spread of HIV in the communities they serve. Such data could be surrogates and indicators of the epidemic, perhaps more direct and more reliable than surveillance of seroprevalence, particularly if coupled with occasional point prevalence surveillance. Infection rates have been sufficiently high in a number of places in the country for sufficiently long to ensure that the effects of increased adult morbidity and mortality will be starting to be felt. Alternatively, where infection rates are still low, these data will be useful to establish baselines. Similarly, initial examination of changing costs in hospital procedures and budgets in the face of increasing HIV prevalence would be valuable indicators to help forecast needs within the health system; cost-benefit and cost-effectiveness analysis, particularly related to prevalence rates,[7] would help identify locations of special urgency, given the constraints on health sector financing.

This chapter reports on a small-scale study conducted to test the viability of this approach, to investigate the most appropriate methodology, and to collect some initial data. This study investigated morbidity and mortality patterns in a selection of hospitals around the country. The experience of working on this, and the data collected, could be the basis for a more substantial, longer-term study of the supply and demand for health care in the context of the epidemic.

6. See the Concept Plan of the National Apical Advisory Committee of the Ministry of Health and Family Welfare, GOI, October 1997.

7. Bloom & Godwin eds: *The Economics of HIV & AIDS; the Case of South and South East Asia,* OUP, 1997.

Study Design: Hospital Morbidity and Mortality Patterns

Premise
The increasing prevalence of HIV in the population will lead to changes in morbidity and mortality rates and patterns in the community. These changes will affect hospital use, occupancy and stay outcomes, and be reflected in hospital morbidity, mortality, and usage patterns.

Objectives
* Establish hospital morbidity and mortality patterns.
* Establish hospital stay and outcome patterns.
* Identify changes in these over time, and the reasons for any changes.

Data required
Admissions: age/sex/origin (place)/ illness
Stay: duration
Outcome: discharge/ death/etc.
(?) Previous admission history
(?) Catchment population/environment: population, population change, etc.

Method
Review and analyse discharge and admission records.

The Study at the TB Hospital

An initial trial of the methodology was conducted at the Rajan Babu TB Hospital in Delhi. In this first trial, data from the hospital's Annual Reports for the eleven years 1986–96 were analysed. These records were detailed and accurate, and easily accessible. The results showed a remarkable stability and consistency in admission patterns (Figure 1).

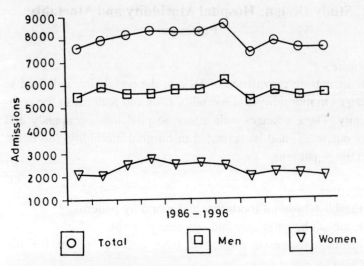

FIGURE 1: RB TB Hospital: Admissions.

Discussions with the hospital staff, however, suggested that the relatively unchanging patterns are likely to be the result of the hospital operating under great pressure and at maximum bed occupancy. An attempt was therefore made to identify some specific items within the data set which might be sensitive to changes in patterns in the catchment area in spite of the very high demand for beds. Figure 2 shows one set of age- and sex-specific admissions.

It is suggested that the tendency of HIV infection to cluster among younger adults should produce a shift in age-specific admissions.[8] TB incidence has been shown to move towards younger adults as HIV prevalence increases. Any significant trend towards younger admissions would therefore be highly suggestive of increasing HIV prevalence rates. Similarly, Figure 3 shows death rates for the last 11 years. These again might be sensitive to increasing HIV prevalence; HIV infection increases

_____

8.   J.P. Narain, M.C. Raviglione, & A. Kochi: 'HIV-associated tuberculosis in developing countries: epidemiology and strategies for prevention', *Tubercle and Lung Disease*, 73, 311–21, 1992.

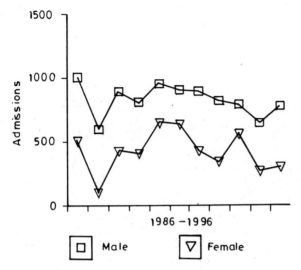

FIGURE 2: RB TB Hospital: Admissions 15–24 years.

mortality rates among TB infected patients. It is interesting to note, but perhaps of no statistical significance as yet, that death rates for female admissions are generally catching up with those for males in the last few years, suggesting an increasing number of acutely ill females being admitted.

Further Data Collection and Analysis

Since the initial investigation at the TB hospital had been so rewarding, it was decided to sample a few other hospitals to see what could be found.

Khurda and Balipatana Hospitals in Orissa
Data were collected from Khurda and Balipatana hospitals in Orissa. Some interesting patterns can be seen. In Khurda: while total admissions remain fairly stable, female admissions have largely overtaken male admissions: from 46 per cent of all admissions in 1986 to 53 per cent in 1996 (Figure 4). In addition, death rates (annual deaths as a percentage of admissions) for both sexes have steadily climbed in the last decade (from 8 per cent for both

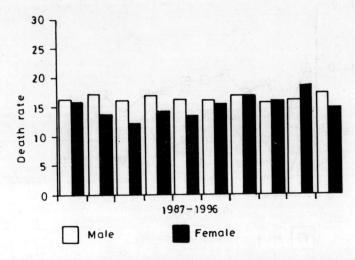

FIGURE 3: RB TB Hospital: Death rate (deaths as % admissions).

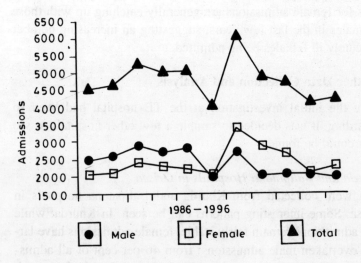

FIGURE 4: Khurda Hospital, Orissa: Admissions.

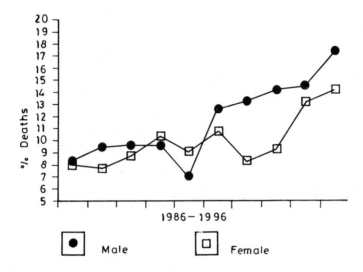

FIGURE 5: Khurda Hospital, Orissa: Death rates.

sexes in 1986 to 14 per cent for women and 18 per cent for men in 1996–Figure 5). Finally, there seems to have been a fairly steep rise in TB admissions in the hospital—annual TB cases have nearly doubled between 1986 and 1996 (Figure 6).

There could be many reasons for these changes in pattern in Khurda Hospital: changes in staffing and services provided (e.g. more maternity care). or declining budgets and availability of drugs or changes in the health of the community around. These data do not offer any hint of the reasons but they do present a fairly consistent pattern, which is certainly worth investigating. It would be very interesting to discover, for example, whether the significant rise in death rates from about 1991 onwards was the result of increasing numbers of acute infections in unrecognised HIV positive patients, arising from the return of HIV-infected migrant workers from Mumbai, Calcutta, Delhi or Chennai.

In Balipatana female admissions are consistently two to three times male admissions (Figure 7). But here the investigation failed. It was not possible, in terms of the pilot study, to get

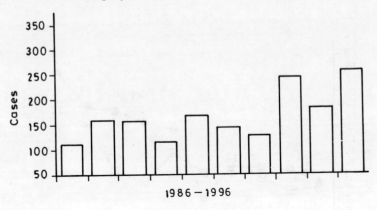

FIGURE 6: Khurda Hospital, Orissa: Annual TB cases.

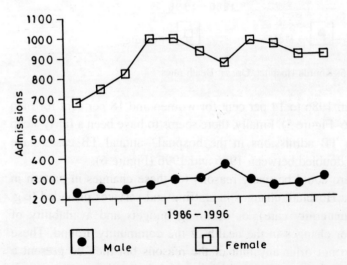

FIGURE 7: Balipatana Hospital, Orissa; Admissions.

accurate and consistent sex- and age-specific admission figures, and death rates.

Kalawati Saran, SSK and Safdarjung Hospitals, Delhi
Further data were collected at three hospitals in Delhi. Kalawati Saran, the paediatric wing of Lady Hardinge Medical College with an admission rate of 450 beds; SSK, an 800 bedded hospital,

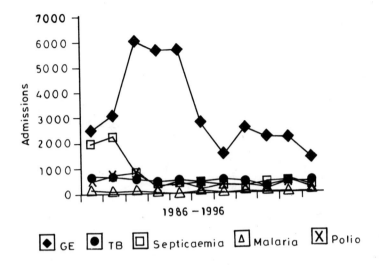

FIGURE 8: KS Hospital: Paediatric admissions by illness.

formerly for women only, attached to Lady Hardinge Medical College; and Safdarjung Hospital, one of the largest in New Delhi. Again, some interesting baseline data emerge.

Figures 8 and 9 show the fairly static pattern of admissions over the last ten years at the paediatric and SSK hospitals. Note that at SSK all obstetric and gynaecological admissions have been excluded from these data; the preponderance of TB is noticeable here. Figure 10 shows the stability of death rates (deaths as a percentage of admissions) at the women's and children's hospitals. The much higher death rates among children is startling. It is likely that death rates, measured in this way, could be a very useful monitoring indicator. There is some evidence[9] that deaths rates show an initial increase at the first impact of acutely ill HIV positive patients who start being admitted in large numbers. Figure 11 shows the major increase in TB at the Safdarjung hospital.

9. Floyd & Gilks, op. cit.

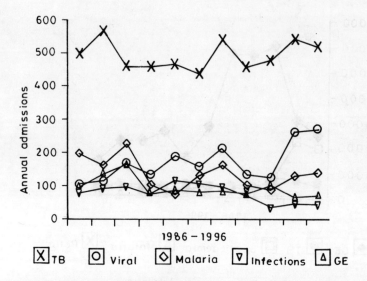

FIGURE 9: SSK Hospital: Kinds of Illness.

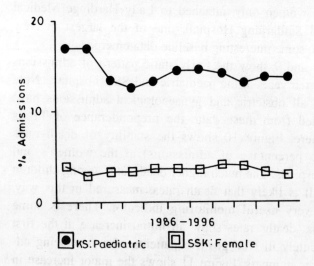

FIGURE 10: Death rates (deaths as % admissions).

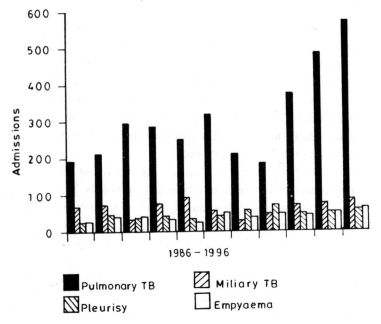

FIGURE 11: Safdarjung Hospital: TB admissions.

Comments and Conclusions

It must be pointed out that the terms of this pilot study did not allow for the testing of the statistical validity of any of these data; that would have to wait for a more focused, in-depth study. This pilot study was merely to determine the availability of such data, and whether their collection would be easy, and would suggest significant patterns. This has clearly been demonstrated.

By and large, it appears that, within Delhi at least, few changes in morbidity and mortality, as reflected in the hospital admissions studied, have occurred so far—with the exception of the increase in TB in Safdarjung Hospital. Given what is known of the prevalence of HIV in the country this is not surprising. This study has generated a clear baseline, however, by which changes over the next few years can be monitored. It has also demonstrated the relative ease with which hospital data can be collected and analysed.

One problem area in future work along these lines, however, is the extent to which the morbidity and mortality changes expected to occur as a result of the spread of HIV will in fact be reflected in public sector hospitals. On the one hand, a very great deal of medical care in India is provided by the private sector; on the other, HIV infection may be spreading most among the poor, who are most likely to use public sector hospitals. This is an area requiring considerable further study.

A second thing to note in further work will be whether the changes in morbidity patterns to be expected will be large enough to be reflected in overall hospital admission statistics, or whether they will be lost in the normal variations that our data show in such enormous hospitals, with such high patient turnovers. It may be necessary to look in considerably more detail at specific age groups, at sample periods (e.g. admissions over a one week period), or at specific kinds of admissions (e.g. TB among women).

Studies, such as these, both with respect to their methodologies and their results, can be important policy tools for decision-makers. They can:

- provide simple baselines to monitor changes in the pattern of disease (e.g. function as part of the surveillance system for TB, HIV, etc.);
- help identify admission patterns which can be used to allocate resources more efficiency within the health system (e.g. identify hospitals or clinics which will face additional burdens of disease arising from increasing HIV prevalence in particular catchment areas or among particular catchment populations);
- provide a mechanism for identifying changing priorities for resource allocation (e.g. training, drugs, management routines, etc.) within hospitals.

These studies need to be replicated in a wide range of hospitals, in various parts of the country.

CHAPTER SIX

HIV Infection in the Workforce and its Perceived Impact on Industry

SUBHASH HIRA, SWATI GUPTA AND PETER GODWIN

The India Labour Force and the HIV Epidemic

According to the 1991 Census the Indian workforce comprised 37.7 per cent of the total population: 314 million workers; 35.6 per cent of the male population and 22.7 per cent of the female. The vast majority of this workforce (59 per cent) are engaged in agriculture and allied activities. An additional 15 per cent are employed in small businesses; 8.5 per cent work in the organised sector, such as mining and manufacturing; and 17.7 per cent work in the service sector. The extent of child labour is quite unclear; certainly, however, tens of millions of children work as well.

At present the HIV epidemic is unevenly distributed in terms of geographic location and socio-economic levels. High prevalences of infection are reported from metropolitan and large cities, and expanding, industrial peri-urban areas. In Chapter 3 of this volume (Eliot), prevalence levels between 2 per cent and 3 per cent are reported for Thane and Ahmednagar outside Mumbai. Anecdotal evidence suggests that prevalence is high within the lower (unskilled) levels of the workforce, and rising steadily among skilled workers, professionals, and managers, in that order. Two industries in Mumbai, for example, offer voluntary, anonymous HIV counselling and testing services for their employees. The prevalence of HIV infection in 1996 was 3 per cent in one of these and 2.5 per cent in the other. (Both industries offered testing to workers based within the factory).[1] This is likely to have a selection bias skewing prevalence towards the lower side because of confidentiality concerns on the part of workers taking the HIV test.

Since HIV primarily affects sexually active adults (15–49 years), who also comprise the main bulk of the workforce, it is evident that ill-health and death due to this epidemic will affect businesses.

The incidence of HIV among the workforce is dependent upon several factors. The most important probably are: an epidemiological 'pool' of HIV infections (among commercial sex workers, for example); the prevalence of multi-partner sex activity, or other 'risk behaviour'; prevalence of STDs; and rate of condom use. While overall HIV prevalence rates in India are low, they are rising rapidly in the particular environments in which the bulk of the workforce lives and works, and where the conditions described above are favourable for the spread of HIV. For example, the prevalence of HIV among commercial sex workers in Mumbai increased from 51 per cent in 1993 to an estimated 60 per cent in 1996. By comparison, it rose from 0.5 per cent in 1986 to 34.5 per cent in 1990 in Vellore. Among women attending antenatal clinics (usually regarded as a marker for the general adult population), prevalence had reached 2.5 per cent in Mumbai and 2.0 per cent in Tirupati by 1994.[2]

Studies of industrial labour in Madras (DESH,[3] ILO[4]), Delhi, and Mumbai (CORT[5]) and of transportation workers in Bengal

---

1.   ARCON, personal communication.

2.   Shiv Lal & B.B. Thakur: 'The Problem of HIV and AIDS in India', *Current Science*, Vol. 69, No. 10, Nov. 1995.

3.   Unpublished study by Deepam Educational Society for Health, commissioned by the UNDP Regional HIV Project, New Delhi, 1994 (mimeo).

4.   Unpublished study by Employers Federation of South India, commissioned by ILO, New Delhi, 1995 (mimeo).

5.   Unpublished study by Centre for Operations Research and Training, commissioned by the UNDP Regional HIV Project, New Delhi, 1994/5 (mimeo).

and in the Indian Railways (UNDP[6]) confirm a significant level of risk behaviour amongst the labour force. These studies fairly consistently record that some 20–25 per cent of workers indulge in multi-partner sex (whether with formal commercial sex workers or with 'friends'), with condom use rates in these encounters under 5 per cent. Since these figures are based on self-reported behaviour, they can be expected to be significantly under-reported. Indeed, in the ILO study in Madras, while 25 per cent of the workers interviewed said they themselves visited commercial sex workers, 54 per cent reported that their colleagues did so. The UNDP Railways study calculated that given the prevalence of this kind of risk behaviour, and the prevalence of HIV in the country, by the year 2000, 6 per cent of all railway employees are likely to be HIV positive. Surveys of truck-drivers in Calcutta and Kashmir confirmed seropositivity rates in 1993/94 of 7–10 per cent.[7]

Another factor that is conventionally associated with a higher level of risk behaviour is migration for employment, and consequent lack of access to spousal sex. The CORT study found that among migrant workers in Mumbai and Delhi, those living with their families were half as likely to report going to CSWs as those not staying with their families. In Delhi, those who visited their families more frequently were less likely to visit CSWs. This study revealed that 46 per cent of workers in Mumbai and 65 per cent in Delhi, were migrants. Of these, approximately 20 per cent were living alone; in addition, 26 per cent in Delhi and 56 per cent in Mumbai were from a distant state. Consequently, HIV prevalence is likely to rise rapidly among the migrant workforce.

At the levels of unprotected multi-partner sex already noted, there is significant likelihood of HIV spreading amongst industrial workers as HIV prevalence rates continue to rise in the environment.

---

6. Unpublished study commissioned by UNDP, New Delhi, 1994 (mimeo).

7. Asha Rao, Moni Nag, Kingshuk Mishra & Arati Dey: 'Sexual Behaviour Pattern of Truck Drivers and their Helpers in relation to Female Sex Workers', *The Indian Journal of Social Work,* October, 1994.

The Distribution of Infection Within the Workforce

Much less is currently known about the distribution (present or likely) of HIV infection within the labour force—though there are some indicators. Predicting this distribution and its effects has two elements: identifying whether particular categories of employees are likely to be more vulnerable or more at risk, and whether infection with HIV among particular categories is likely to have more impact on the business. A study in Kenya, for example, calculated that while technical professional staff represented on an average only 3 per cent of employees in companies studied, they would account for more than 20 per cent of costs arising from HIV/AIDS, presumably assuming that HIV infection was distributed evenly across all categories of employees.[8] Were HIV to occur more in that small group, these costs would be even higher.

Some elements that might affect this distribution have been noted in the studies in India so far. Both the DESH study and the ILO study in Madras found that the tendency towards risk behaviour (primarily the tendency to purchase commercial sex) varied. The ILO study found that this tendency was greater among older, more educated employees, and those with higher incomes; the DESH study found it greater among older employees and those earning more, though not necessarily more educated—suggesting the skilled artisan, often a critical member of the labour force.

Analysis of hospital-based data collected on 3520 persons referred to the AIDS Research & Control Centre (ARCON) at J.J. Hospital in Mumbai between April 1994 and June 1996 revealed that 27 per cent of males, and 18 per cent of females who tested HIV positive had completed high school or higher education. Of the HIV-positive males, 41 per cent were engaged in skilled work, while 68 per cent of the HIV positive females were housewives. Assuming that the referral of persons on the

---

8.   Steven Forsythe et al. eds: *AIDS in Kenya*, USAID/FHI/AIDSCAP, 1996.

basis of clinical suspicion of immune suppression was unbiased, mapping was done for the city of Mumbai using HIV density ratios for geographic locations. The highest HIV density ratios were obtained for suburbs representing middle-class residential, and industrial zones of the city. While this study reconfirms the uneven geographic distribution of HIV in Mumbai, it does make clear that the epidemic has spread to populations which traditionally have had a low perception of their vulnerability to this epidemic.

But this raises a further set of issues: how do businesses respond to illness and death among their employees? The common reaction among many business men is based on the assumption that only 'crude' basic labour are at risk; since these are in surplus throughout the country, business men assume that they will easily absorb the impact of increases in deaths and absenteeism because of illness among casual labour. But if this assumption is incorrect, and if infections are evenly distributed, or even predominate among the better paid, the skilled, etc., absorbing this impact will be less easy. As the Kenya data quoted above show, a small number of sick higher level employees can be very expensive to businesses; even more worrying, while casual labour may be in surplus in India, skilled and managerial labour is often in short supply. Illness and deaths among such levels could be very expensive to businesses in terms of replacement, recruitment, and training costs. Particularly important here is the kind of benefits that businesses have for employees.

Data from Zambia[9] and Uganda[10] show that costs associated with illness (medical care, medicines, etc) are more important than costs associated with death. This has two dimensions: most businesses tend to make more generous provision for employees who are sick than for those who die; second, people living with HIV tend to have a series of episodes of illness and incapacitation before they die.

---

9. *The effects of HIV/AIDS on farming systems in eastern Africa,* FAO, 1995.
10. *The Hidden Cost of AIDS.* PANOS Institute, 1992.

Discussions with employers suggest a number of practices with regard to health and welfare benefits in the private sector, ranging from absolutely none, through a variety of reimbursement schemes for medical expenses incurred, to 'company clinics', in-house health services, and full health insurance. The CORT study, for example, found that 38 per cent of workers in Delhi but only 12 per cent in Mumbai had some form of medical insurance, most of which (86 per cent in Delhi and 65 per cent in Mumbai) was ESIS (Employees State Insurance Scheme); for the rest, roughly half (46 per cent in Delhi and 59 per cent in Mumbai) got reimbursed, most with a fixed amount, and a small percentage for actual expenditure. Unfortunately these data were not disaggregated by category of worker.

What *does* emerge from this review, however, is the potential for a severe impact on the private sector in India. While many workers are not covered for benefits, so that employers are unlikely to incur significant expenditure on their illness or death, a very significant proportion are. Serious increases in this expenditure will have to be met from somewhere. In addition, if, as some of the data suggest, more skilled employees (and thus employees more difficult to replace) are at higher risk, companies' costs could rise significantly. A study of 33 businesses in Zambia revealed an increased crude annual mortality rate from 0.25 in 1985 to 1.83 in 1993 (*p*-value 0.001). The number of employees in these companies remained the same. During the same period AIDS deaths increased from 1 to 36 while deaths due to unknown causes increased from 14 to 286.[11]

As Giraud suggests, these kinds of costs to employers get handled in one (or all) of three ways: passed on to consumers, in increased prices; passed on to the public sector, through refusal to accept them; or taken out of profits.[12] All three responses signify

11. F. Baggaley et al.: 'Impact of HIV infection on Zambian businesses', *British Medical Journal* 309:1549–50, 1994.

12. Patrick Giraud: 'The Economic Impact of AIDS at the Sectoral Level; Developing an Assessment Methodology and Applying it to Thailand's Transport Sector' in *Economic Implications of AIDS in Asia*, D. Bloom & J. Lyons, eds. UNDP, New Delhi, 1993.

a lowering of productivity. While this is theoretically clear, how has business in fact responded?

The Response of Industry in Mumbai

Professionals who know or work with AIDS awareness programmes with industries in several cities of India acknowledge that industry has displayed only a 'knee-jerk' response and is still not convinced of the real medical and socio-economic impact of the epidemic. Obviously, decision-makers are looking for more convincing surveillance figures.

To attempt to understand better what industry thinks, a knowledge, attitude and practice (KAP) study was conducted in Mumbai by two of the authors in 1996 with the participation of seven locally-owned companies, each having a workforce of more than 5,000 (see Table 1). These industries were involved in textiles (2), petrochemicals (2), automobiles (2) and machine manufacture (1). At each industry, efforts were made to obtain two key respondents in each of the following categories to respond to a structured questionnaire: senior manager (13), mid-level manager (14), supervisor (14), union leader (7), and medical officer (14). The salient findings of the KAP study involving a total of 62 respondents were as follows:

- Almost a third of the respondents representing all seven companies had personally known a co-worker with HIV/AIDS.
- All companies required a medical examination as part of pre-employment procedure for all levels of workers.
- Out of 62 respondents, 52 rated themselves as 'very' or 'fairly' knowledgeable about HIV/AIDS.
- Misconceptions such as transmission of HIV by mosquito could be cultural because of this vector's association with malaria which is holoendemic in India.
- None of the companies had written policies or guidelines regarding employees with HIV/AIDS.

TABLE 1: Knowledge, Attitude and Practice (KAP) study among respondents of 7 industries in Mumbai

Knowledge (n=62)

1.	Adequate General AIDS knowledge relating to epidemiology and disease progression	55
2.	Misconceptions such as:	
	a. Mosquito transmission of HIV	12
	b. Sharing cups and dishes can transmit HIV	5
	c. Hugging someone who has HIV can transmit HIV	4
	d. Healthy-looking HIV positive person cannot transmit	3
	e. AIDS can be cured if detected early	16
3.	Who should be involved in developing of HIV/AIDS policy in the company?	
	a. Personnel/HRD	47
	b. Medical department	47
	c. Labour Unions	27
	d. Medical advisory group	24
	e. CEO/Chairman/President	15
4.	Direct experience of employees with HIV/AIDS	
	a. Knew about an employee who tested HIV positive	29
	b. Personally knew someone in the workforce who tested HIV positive	25
	c. Knew about an employee who had AIDS	26
	d. Personally knew someone in the workforce who had AIDS	22
	e. Knew of an employee who died with AIDS	24
	f. Personally knew someone in the workforce who died with AIDS	19
	g. Knew family member or a member of household of an employee who tested HIV positive	9

Attitude (n=62)

5.	Company management concerned about AIDS	44
6.	Employees concerned about AIDS	33
7.	Issues	
	a. Company should institute HIV testing of current employees	20
	b. Test results should be given both to employee and employer	48

(Contd.)

TABLE 1: Contd.

c. Most employees will not be resistant to work alongside an employee with HIV/AIDS	34
8. AIDS will increase cost of company's medical expenses in 5 years	34
9. Company should pay for treatment of an employee with HIV/AIDS	47
10. Employees will favour company participation in AIDS education programmes	50
Practice (n=7 companies)	
11. HIV/AIDS activities. Number of companies providing:	
a. Distribution of condoms to employees	2
b. STD diagnosis/treatment	3
c. Voluntary testing/counselling services	2
12. Companies considering setting up HIV/AIDS programme	7
13. Number of companies rejecting an applicant testing HIV positive at pre-employment	4
14. Number of companies supplementing disability payments for an employee with AIDS	5

- Most senior managers did not support labour unions, boards of directors, or medical consultants for HIV advice, nor did they favour drawing on the practices of other companies that might already have written policies. They preferred that for developing HIV/AIDS policies for their companies, the task be assigned to their own Human Resource Development and Medical departments.

- Most respondents were not aware whether or not medical expenses of their companies had increased due to employees with HIV/AIDS.

- Three-quarters of the respondents, belonging to all the seven companies, felt that the company should pay the medical expenses of employees with HIV/AIDS.

- None of the companies admitted to altering their hiring, promotion, or firing policies on the basis of their concerns about HIV/AIDS in the workforce.

- The senior management (10 out of 13) and union leaders overwhelmingly felt that their companies would get involved with
the AIDS problem if many more of their employees got AIDS,
if employees pushed for it, if productivity was suffering, or if
employee morale was affected by HIV/AIDS in the workforce.
- The respondents' support for appeals by community leaders,
celebrities, or government officials was extremely low. By
comparison, appeals by members of AIDS organisations were
rated higher by all respondents.
- There was overwhelming support from managers and union
respondents for continued employment of employees with
HIV/AIDS.

Very little information was available on practices because
most respondents had not yet been involved in major decisions
such as those concerning long-term care, co-worker issues,
home-based care etc.

While adequate knowledge and positive attitudes therefore appear to exist among representatives of all categories of the
workforce, appropriate policies and guidelines have not been for-
mulated so far. Decision-makers are not convinced of the need to
act. There is, therefore, an urgent need to strengthen surveillance
to generate reliable data on the level of HIV infection in the
community and the workforce and its likely implications; to in-
itiate well-designed operational research to demonstrate the impact of the epidemic on the micro-economics of the business; and
to institute intervention programmes.

* * *

Discussion: The Personal Face of the Epidemic

S: As you well know, Peter, I was discriminated against in two 'work force'
situations. So I feel very strongly about this.

PG: Yes, I do know. But tell me about it.

S: As is often the case, I was initially tested for HIV on the grounds of a
'Pre-employment' medical check-up; and my employment was forfeited on the

grounds of HIV status. The reason I was given was the 'policy' (or, when I asked for clarification, the 'lack of policy') by management in 'situations such as this'.

PG: What you mean by 'lack of policy' is that they hadn't been told specifically by management that they could hire someone who was HIV positive, nor that they couldn't. And in the absence of specific instructions they basically discriminated: it was safest not to hire you?

S: Exactly. And this is the problem. It is not always what you might call 'positive discrimination'; it is often a kind of negative avoidance.

PG: Does this only happen at this kind of pre-employment medical screening?

S: Oh, no. In the majority of situations it comes up when people are tested for HIV in businesses by the medical staff, whenever they fall sick. The management is then informed first, if there is an HIV positive result, even before the individual who has been tested. In one public sector concern an individual I know was tested, and was found to be positive. The whole office got to know about his sero-status even before he did! In fact, he found out he was positive when he was about to get into the lift, and the lift operator told him not to enter the lift as he 'had AIDS'!

PG: But in the survey we report in the chapter there seems to be a strong sense of support for people who are HIV positive.

S: Well, the private sector speaks quite 'supportively' in public, but responds in quite the opposite way when it comes to their own workforce. None of the supportive talk counts for much when they are faced with the reality of one of their own staff or workers being HIV positive. When the word gets around, employers and employees alike are panic-stricken. 'His presence will affect our business' is the common reaction by employers. It is worse with the employees. People don't want to associate with him (though there are exceptions). Most people will say that they are uncomfortable working with an HIV positive employee. People are over-reactive when it comes to 'AIDS'. Most often the employers want to terminate the staff member on the grounds of 'inefficiency'; or give him long leave with salary, which will be sent to his residence.

PG: Anything to get him out of the way; to hide him.

S: Yes; but it is not simple. Although most employers want to simply dismiss a worker who is HIV positive, there are others who are not so direct; they want to 'transfer' him to a place where he will not have 'so much strain'; or where his confidentiality can be protected, or he can have a 'special placement' so that his health is not compromised. In all these responses it is really a case of trying to hide him!

PG: Then the idea of just accepting sero-status openly, and refusing to allow any discrimination of any sort, for or against, is not common?

S: No.

CHAPTER SEVEN

The Epidemic in Rural Communities: The Relevance of the African Experience for India

TONY BARNETT[1]

Introduction

The concepts of susceptibility to the epidemic (the likelihood and socio-economic parameters of rapid growth of infections) and vulnerability to the longer-term social and economic impacts of the epidemic, when applied to India, suggest a significantly different pattern of both epidemic development and of long-term social and economic impact to that observed in Africa. This observation is tied in particular to the density of population and the frequency of population movement between rural and urban areas. The result is that urban and rural seroprevalence and case rates might be expected to move closer to each other over a shorter period than has been the case in Africa.

1. This chapter was prepared with assistance from many individuals, all of whom it is not possible to thank individually. Fieldwork in Rajasthan and some of the ideas in the report were considerably assisted by the hard work of, and discussions with, four foreign volunteers working at Seva Mandir who spent time with me in some villages in rural Rajasthan. They are: Ilona Barratt, Peter Harrison, Russell Hartenstine and Snehal Shah. In addition, the assistance, ideas and advice of Apoor Christopher Bishwas and Mahesh Acharya who acted as interpreters were also of the greatest possible help. Special thanks are due to the staff of Seva Mandir in Udaipur who extended excellent facilities and made me feel very welcome in their busy organisation. In particular, thanks to the Chief Executive of Seva Mandir, Mr Ajay Mehta and to its Medical Director, Dr Lodha. Of course, none of the above, nor any other informant bears any responsibility for errors of fact or of interpretation. Those are mine alone.

This chapter examines some of the socio-economic elements underlying this analysis, based, as a micro-example, on short field observations in villages around Udaipur, in Rajasthan, and compares these to the experience of a number of countries in east, central and southern Africa.

The extent of climatic dryness and resulting labour bottlenecks is a major element in determining the vulnerability of labour-intensive rural livelihood strategies to the loss of labour to an epidemic disease with cohort-specific morbidity and mortality such as that associated with HIV/AIDS. Comparison of African material with that collected in Rajasthan suggests that the problem in India is likely to differ from that in Africa. In the latter, labour is the main constraint confronting some farming systems in the drier areas, whereas in India, the main constraint is less likely to be labour and more likely to be irrigated land. In fact, evidence from Rajasthan suggests that many rural people are already so poor as a result of shortage of irrigated land or in some cases of any land, that they are already pursuing livelihood strategies which might define them better as 'rural wage labourers' rather than 'subsistence farmers'. This factor, with its resultant frequent population movements between rural and urban areas, is important in the possibly more rapid equalisation of rural and urban rates of infection.

Susceptibility to the Spread of the Disease

The epidemic has a particular 'shape' in each society. So these comments are intended to provide some initial indication of the idea of the way that societies appear to have differential susceptibility to the spread of the disease. Such a concept is not only analytically useful, but should in addition have practical implications. The regions of Africa to which reference has been made are now probably in the fifteenth or even twentieth year of the epidemic. It is therefore possible to look back over this history and ask, 'had we known then what we know now, how and where would we have intervened so as to reduce the rate and extent of propagation of the epidemic?'. It is in answer to this question that some of what follows will endeavour to build on the 'African experience'.

It is necessary to say a word about the relevance or otherwise of 'Africa's' experience of the HIV/AIDS epidemic for 'India'. The inverted commas in the preceding sentence require some explanation. First of all they are necessary because there is no one 'African' experience of HIV/AIDS—the continent south of the Sahara exhibiting considerable diversity; and furthermore, 'India' itself exhibits at least as much diversity as 'Africa'—save for some very important and significant facts: its being a single political entity, its high level of urbanisation, and perhaps also its higher level of industrialisation as compared to most parts of Africa outside of the Republic of South Africa.

Thus each society's HIV/AIDS epidemic will differ in its particulars, reflecting aspects of the cultural, social, economic, and political life of that country. The different aspects of susceptibility and vulnerability in each society are thus weighted differently, and combine, reinforce, and counterbalance each other. The following sections look at some of the more common elements of vulnerability and susceptibility, and, drawing on the African experience and some data from Rajasthan, attempt to suggest some of the ways India may be susceptible and vulnerable.

Political, Economic, Social and Cultural Factors

Two examples from Africa can be considered to illustrate some of the critical political, economic, social, and cultural factors contributing to susceptibility and vulnerability. In Uganda (one of the first and most severely affected countries in Africa), there appear to be specific features which have shaped that epidemic. Notably these include the fact that women have no independent access to land, that there has been a long history of civil unrest and, at times, open warfare in many parts of the country since the early

1970s, and that as a result central government has at times been ineffective and, when not ineffective, often arbitrary. The implications of this for the 'shape' of the epidemic have probably been to increase the rate and direction of its spread as illicit trade, warfare and civil disruption—together with the fact that an east-west trans-African transport route runs across southern Uganda—have interacted to spread the disease into even quite remote areas through a cash–sex nexus in which women with few resources and, most importantly, lacking independent access to land, have exchanged sexual favours for survival or a share in the material benefits of illicit and legal trade or other enterprise.

In Zambia, economy and society have long been shaped in relation to a dominant mining industry fed by long-term labour migration with urban life supported by the artificially priced maize production in the countryside. Here the epidemic's spread and impact may be expected to be greatly influenced by the close and deep links between urban and rural areas through the tradition of labour migration.

In India, rural–urban migration and the particular shape it takes, as well as the mobility of much of India's population, may prove to be an important element in determining particular aspects of India's epidemics. According to the 1981 census, 35 per cent of males and 42 per cent of females in the total population were lifetime migrants. While much of this reflects movements within districts and states (and particularly, in the case of women, migration, on marriage, to the husband's village), 20 per cent of males and 10 per cent of females had moved between states, with 50 per cent of this among men being for employment.

The duration of migration is also critical in India. According to the 1981 census, 10 per cent of inter-regional migrants were resident for less than one year while nearly 60 per cent were resident for more than 10 years, suggesting that migration is a simple affair of moving to the city. Yet more specifically, a study of migrants from 56 villages in Bihar found that 10 per cent migrated for less than three months; 47 per cent for between four and six months; and only 16 per cent for more than 10 months.[2] This suggests a far greater pattern of mobility.

Population Density and Rural-urban Links

An important area of comparison between the African and Indian experience must revolve around the related issues of population density, comparative levels of urbanisation, and the nature of rural–urban relationships. One of the first things in rural areas that strikes a visitor to India who is familiar with Africa is the difference attached to the meaning of the word 'remote'. While in the African context, 'remote' may mean that a settlement is a day or more's walk from a road, or that at least can only be approached by road with some difficulty, this is much less the case in either Rajasthan or Bihar, for example. In addition, population density is just that much greater in India as compared with Africa. India's population density is well over 200 persons per square kilometre; with the exception of Rwanda and Burundi, no East or Central African country has a population density of over 100 persons per square kilometre, and most are below 50.[3]

Were these two factors not in themselves significant, there is a third factor which is of importance. Despite the great poverty of so many of its people, India does have both a primary and secondary industrial base as well as labour-demanding large-scale agriculture. It is not that Africa lacks these things entirely, rather that they exist at a different order of magnitude. There are frequent and varied interactions between town and countryside in India. Here it is not only a matter of the long-term male migration to a few labour demanding large-scale enterprises as it is in Africa. Rather it consists of both large-scale long-term migration to urban centres as well as shorter duration, in some cases daily, commuting from villages as much as 15 or 20 kilometres from cities and large towns in search of labouring work.

2. P.P. Ghosh, Alakh A. Sharma: 'Seasonal Migration of Rural Labour in Bihar', *Labour and Development,* July–December, 1995.
3. World Development Report, OUP. 1993.

These close and frequent links between rural and urban areas, much closer and much more frequent than is generally the case in Africa, would seem to indicate that in the Indian case one might expect the rate of transmission from urban to rural areas to be more rapid than in Africa and thus for the difference between rural and urban rates of seroprevalence to assume a less steep gradient over a shorter period. In other words, the movement towards equality between urban and rural rates in India should be more rapid than has been the case in Africa. At present it is, of course, impossible to make any empirically informed statement as to what these rates may in general be; though even in heavily burdened environments (e.g. Rakai, Uganda) urban rates of 20 per cent in the 15–50 age group are matched by rural rates of less than 10 per cent.

Sexual Culture and Sexual Health

In addition to these economic, political, and social factors, there may be others which are specific to the African situation. The list that follows must be treated with extreme caution and risks homogenising what has already been noted to be a highly differentiated entity. Among these factors, some of which may or may not be specific to Africa, are: some sexual cultures which are apparently more relaxed than those stated publicly to be the case in India and which approximate to the northern European pattern (but we should note that we know very little empirically about the reality of sexual cultures and networks); high levels of STD illness which may constitute co-factors in infection; generally poor health status of many populations in Africa together with the presence of large numbers of opportunistic infections; the presence in some parts of Africa (but it must be emphasised not in all, and certainly not necessarily in the earliest infected areas) of sexual practices (notably 'dry sex' in some cultures), which it is sometimes argued may enhance viral transmission through increased minor genital laceration (and the question of whether similar or other practices are entirely absent in India); the claim (by John Caldwell[4]) that in Africa one may discern a differential distribution of rates of infection as between societies which do and do not practise male circumcision, with the circumcised being less prone to infection (in which case it would be necessary to consider how or whether this factor is of importance in the Indian context, given that male circumcision is also practised by some communities and not by others).

An authoritative survey of what is known about the sexual culture of India is in Moni Nag's book, *'Sexual behaviour and AIDS in India'*.[5] Nag reports on a number of studies of sexual attitudes among various groups. In a large survey of college students and young graduates in 16 cities the conservative concept of premarital sex as sin is held only by 23 per cent of the men and 10 per cent of the women.[6] The fact that 40 per cent of the men and 33 per cent of the women disagreed with the statement that it is a sin to have premarital sex contradicts the stereotype belief commonly held by a large section of the Indian population. Perhaps more surprising is the fact that 16 per cent of the men and 5 per cent of the women were radical enough to agree with the statement that both young men and women must have sex before marriage. A remarkable shift from the traditional condemnation of premarital sex both among men and women is also revealed in a substantial percentage of men (46 per cent) and women (44 per cent) agreeing with the statement that having premarital sex is the concern of the individual and not of society. Another study of 300 men diagnosed as having a sexually transmitted disease in the STD clinic of Lucknow hospital in 1976, found that 81 per cent had premarital sexual experience. Illiteracy was high (37 per

---

4. J.C. Caldwell & P. Caldwell: 'The nature and limits of the Sub-Saharan African AIDS epidemic: evidence from geographic and other patterns', *Population and Development Review*, Vol. 19, No. 4, 817–48, December 1993.

5. Moni Nag: *Sexual Behavour and AIDS in India*, Vikas Publishing House, New Delhi, 1996.

6. Conducted by the Family Planning Association of India.

cent) among the respondents: 35 per cent had education up to high school or above.[7]

A final observation concerning the differences between Africa and India has to do with polygyny—either simultaneous or serial. In both Muslim and non-Muslim Africa, polygyny is quite widespread (although probably not as widespread as some outside observers have assumed). In India, the possibilities for this are quite limited and it is understood that it does not occur among Hindu communities. It is, however, said to be practised by both Muslims and also by tribal peoples. Much else is said by non-tribal people concerning the sexual lives of tribal peoples: they are relaxed in their sexual mores, they practise polygyny both simultaneous and serial. How far this is the case is not known to the present writer. However, what is important to note is that whatever the truth of such accounts they can become the stuff of stigmatisation and victimisation. If tribal people are also poor (which they often are) and thus, as experience elsewhere has shown, perhaps more susceptible to infection, then it is very important that their particular sexual behaviours and practices should not become part of a further stigmatising mythology. What the practical implications of polygyny are for the propagation of the epidemic is not clear. In Africa, there have been few suggestions that polygyny alone has been a significant factor on its own. It is only significant within the wider cultural and social context within which it is practised.[8] The evidence for this view (and it is only a view and the evidence is very limited and is likely to remain so for obvious reasons of sensitivity) is one small

---

7. Vijay Narayan: *Venereal Diseases: A Social Dilemma*, Cosmo Publications, New Delhi 1984.

8. John and Pat Caldwell: 'The social context of AIDS in Sub-Saharan Africa', *Population and Development Review*, Vol. 15, No. 2, 185–234, 1989; 'The Nature and limits of the Sub-Saharan African AIDS epidemic: evidence from geographic and other patterns', *Population and Development Review*, Vol. 19, No. 4, 817–48, 1993; and associated rejoinders by M-N Le Blanc, D. Meintel, V. Piché: 'The African sexual system: comment on Caldwell et al., *Population and Development Review*, 497–505, Vol. 17, September 1991.

survey in Uganda which compared seroprevalence rates in Muslims and non-Muslims and found that the former had a lower prevalence than the latter.[9] On the assumption that the Muslims were more likely to be polygynists and also the men circumcised (no data were collected on these variables), it may be suggested that polygyny is not on its own, a predisposing factor to infection.

Social Security and Civil Society

Perhaps the greatest contrast between the circumstances of India in comparison with those of Africa has to do with the degree of political and social security. This point forms a link between the organising idea of this section and the next. There can be little doubt that effective state organisation is a factor which plays a part in reducing the susceptibility and vulnerability of a society to epidemic spread. Widespread social disruption and insecurity has certainly played a part in the shape of the epidemic in Uganda and also no doubt in some other parts of Africa. This factor seems, by and large, to be absent from the Indian scene, perhaps with the exception of some areas in the north-east of the country, where it is possibly not coincidental that there is a marked IDU problem with associated increased risks of infection. Thus, the higher degree of social security in India as opposed to the situation in Africa might be a factor in reducing societal susceptibility to epidemic spread.

In addition, despite the major role played by the state in India over the last fifty years, it seems never to have occupied the same autonomous, sometimes all-encompassing and abusive role that has all too often been the case in Africa. This (and perhaps other cultural factors) has meant that there exists in India a rich and vibrant civil society, independent of the state. Such a highly developed civil society means that India is better placed to

---

9.   J.W. Carswell, W. Maawali & R. Moser: Unpublished poster presentation 'Can one use simple demographic data to determine low HIV prevalence blood donors in an African city?', IVth International Conference on AIDS and Associated Cancers in Africa, 18 20 October, 1989, Marseilles, France, poster 385.

respond to the vulnerabilities of impact through means and organisations independent of the state and based in local communities. The existence of many indigenous non-governmental organisations is indicative of this capacity.

However, despite these positive features, the sharp contrast between rich and poor in India, and the effective exclusion of the very poor, both rural and urban, from national life may also be seen as a factor which both increases susceptibility to infection and also makes dealing with the long-term impact more difficult. Hence, continuing and sustained efforts to deal with poverty will form a crucial component in the struggle against both susceptibility to infection and vulnerability to the effects of excess morbidity and mortality.

Vulnerability to the Impact of the Epidemic

Vulnerability, in contrast to susceptibility, describes the idea of openness to the impact of the disease—the longer-term social and economic implications of such potentially widespread increases in mortality and morbidity. Two particular aspects are examined in this section: the impact of increased adult mortality on farming systems and livelihoods, and the impact on the household in the form of orphaning and on the elderly.

Labour Intensive Rural Livelihood Strategies

In relation to the experience of 'Africa', of considerable importance is the issue of the sustainability of small-scale, essentially subsistence, labour-intensive rural production—which mainly, but not exclusively, refers to subsistence farming and associated rural livelihood strategies. The relative vulnerability of rural livelihoods and in particular the agricultural element is tied to dryness and the consequent requirement for intensive labour in short periods around the rains in order to establish the crops. These factors, rainfall and the mobilisation of labour—mainly household labour—have a strong effect on range of crops grown, final yields, maintenance of rural infrastructure such as irrigation and terracing works, and thus on the food security of rural households and communities.

In south-western Uganda, rainfall is relatively high and fairly dependable, with one drought year in ten, and has a bimodal distribution.[10] Traditionally this has enabled people to grow a wide range of food crops as well as robusta coffee. In this area, seroprevalence levels have been observed to be high for at least the last eight years. Thus, in some age cohorts (men and women aged 20–30 years), they may reach 30 per cent in small trading centres only ten kilometres from a main road and have been observed at 8–10 per cent in rural communities only a few kilometres from these trading centres. The effects of HIV-related illness and death were observed on rural production in a robust farming system in 1989 and again in 1993. In the first observation, the effect was already becoming apparent with some, mainly poorer, households having to restrict the range of crops grown, reorganise farm-household labour allocations and resort to a range of coping mechanisms including the withdrawal of children (particularly girls) from school, the taking in of orphans, and increased debt to pay for medical expenses. By 1993, the situation in these communities had taken a marked downward turn. The age cohort 20–45 was by now severely under-represented in the population and many households had reduced the range of crops being cultivated by 50 per cent—with suspected (but un-

---

10. For detailed information about the impact of HIV/AIDS on rural livelihoods in Uganda, see T. Barnett & P.M. Blaikie: *AIDS in Africa: its present and future impact,* Belhaven Press, London and Guilford Press, New York, 1992 and second edition 1995. For information about later developments in Uganda as well as on the situation in Zambia and Tanzania, see T. Barnett. *The Impact of HIV/AIDS on Farming Systems and Rural Livelihoods in Uganda, Tanzania and Zambia: a summary of case material,* Report to FAO and UNDP, Rome, February 1994, published in edited and shortened form as T. Barnett & M. Haslwimmer, *The Impact of HIV/AIDS on Farming Systems in East Africa,* FAO, Rome, May 1995.

proved) effects on nutrition. An additional effect has been on livestock, the keeping of which has also declined as a result of sale to finance medical care and funerals and as a result of poor husbandry consequent upon labour shortages.

This example demonstrates that in Africa, even in a robust farming system, the impact of the disease may be severe. An initial survey in Tanzania in 1993 indicated that the least food-secure areas of the country were by and large also the areas with the lowest levels of seroprevalence.[11] The implications of this finding were taken to mean that in that country there might be a small but significant window for responding to potential disruption of the food production system if government and other agencies were prepared and able to plan ahead and develop labour economising responses specific to the farming systems in question.

Ultimately all labour-intensive systems of rural livelihood are vulnerable to the effects of the epidemic, but the precise level of vulnerability will vary with the spatial propagation of the epidemic in relation to the different systems. This point certainly has relevance to the Indian context and will be elaborated on below in a brief discussion of the situation as observed around Udaipur in Rajasthan.

Rural Livelihoods: Rainfall, Soil and Water Around Udaipur

This section provides some limited and very superficial observations concerning some characteristics of rural livelihoods in Rajasthan as they may (*a*) predispose rural communities to infection; (*b*) predispose rural communities to the impacts of the epidemic over the medium term—by which is meant ten to fifteen years. It is based on a limited number of interviews carried out in a few communities through interpreters by the author of

---

11. T. Barnett: *The Impact of HIV/AIDS on Farming Systems and Rural Livelihoods in Uganda, Tanzania and Zambia: a summary of case material,* Report to FAO and UNDP, Rome, February 1994.

this chapter and his four colleagues. The communities are described briefly as follows:

- *Paderi village*: a mixed Patel, Brahmin and Meghwal village about 170 km from Udaipur in Kherwara Block with an associated settlement of tribal people described as Adivasis.
- *Severi village*: an Adivasi (tribal) settlement in the same area as the above.
- *Katchivasti village*: a village populated by Brahmins, Rajputs, Blacksmiths, Jains and Muslims. Like Paderi, it is in Kherwara Block. It is more of a local centre than the other villages, having a bus stopping place.
- *Jhotri village*: a tribal village about a kilometre from Katchivasti.
- *Gel village*: a tribal village in Badgaon Block about 15 km from Udaipur.

In the general area of Udaipur, about 60 per cent of the population is said to be tribal. Thus the ethnic composition of the five villages visited probably provides some indication of the wider situation in this respect.

The first thing that strikes a visitor to this part of Rajasthan is its aridity and the harshness and bareness of the landscape. Rainfall is variously said to be between 600 mm and 642 mm per year, concentrated in the period July–August. At other times, irrigation is usually necessary for effective cultivation. Soils are mainly clay loams with some red loam and are uniformly rather thin, varying between six inches to three feet with rock breaking the surface in places, while in others, on the hillsides, quite small cultivated pockets of soil are surrounded by large areas of rock. On the valley bottoms, soils appear to be the same but are, as might be expected, among the deepest to be found in the area. Only about 18 per cent (about 118,000 ha) of the total land area is cultivated, mainly, one must assume, because it is either too shallow, infertile or—a major constraint—cannot be irrigated.

The second thing that strikes the visitor to this area is the absence of trees—and then he is twice struck when he realises that this region was deeply forested (presumably with acacia and similar drought-resistant species) until about thirty years ago and that tigers were apparently to be seen quite frequently up to that time, an indication that the environment was sufficiently productive to support both the human population and a food chain containing a major carnivore.

What seems to have occurred in this area is that a nomadic or semi-nomadic people has been settled within recent history, while at the same time their land has come under government control. The establishment of settled agriculture and increased population density (the result of natural increase plus in-migration) has meant that greater pressure has been placed on the land both for cultivation, construction, and fuel wood purposes. The result has been the rapid and acute deforestation and thus the stressed environment which may be observed today. To the non-specialist (but a non-specialist who has seen similarly stressed environments in Ethiopia, Eritrea and other dry regions of Africa) this one looks a small step away from the stage at which the top soil begins to slide down the acute gradients in sheet erosion or to form deep gullies where the gradients are less steep. In places, people have built retaining walls along the contours or have planted stands of 'thur' cactus. How effective these measures are is not known. But if they are effective, and if reforestation programmes are effective, it should be noted that such measures depend upon constant and regular inputs of human labour if they are to be adequately maintained. Should human labour ever become in short supply, then maintenance of these structures is likely to occupy a lower place in the prioritisation of labour in relation to perceived necessities of labour use by the rural households. In addition, pressure on the household labour economy, and particularly pressure on women, may result in premature harvesting of any available trees, including those planted for reforestation purposes. Thus, at the most fundamental level of the maintenance of their soil resources, farming systems in this area are likely to be stressed in response to HIV-related death and illness. In addition, the maintenance of wells and larger water control facilities such as anicuts as well as field channels, are also demanding of time and labour.

Perhaps the most significant piece of information in the preceding, when we consider the system's vulnerability to the impact of HIV/AIDS, is the largely unimodal rainfall distribution, restricted to about eight weeks. This, as has been noted above, is suspected to be a fundamental marker of farming system vulnerability. It is also, in an environment where access to irrigation is probably sharply divided between poorer and richer households, likely to mark out clear distinctions in the potential resilience of households in coping with epidemic-related loss of labour.

A general conclusion of this section is that, while there is a range of livelihood strategies operating in this area of Rajasthan, there is little or no evidence that labour shortage itself constitutes a significant constraint to production, either, despite the brevity of the rains, during the planting season or at harvest time. In contrast to Africa, where land is not usually a constraint in rural systems of production, here it is land, and, in particular, irrigated land, which is the main constraint. Some of the wealthier households which were visited reported hiring labour at times of shortage, but reported no difficulty in finding it. However, the majority of households are not solely dependent upon farming, having inadequate land for their needs and having to search for other income-earning occupations—labouring work, locally, in adjacent towns, or at a greater distance (in some cases Kuwait). Among these labouring occupations is, we are told, a degree of commercial sex work by women from these rural communities. Clearly, this is a major source whereby the infection is likely to be transmitted from the highways and urban areas directly to the villages.

Rural Households: Orphans and Their Care

In the most seriously affected areas of Africa, the epidemic has been responsible for very large numbers of orphans—defined, as in India, as children with one or both parents deceased. The numbers are impressive, running into tens of thousands. Hunter's initial work on this issue in Uganda in 1990 is sufficiently methodologically sound to give credence to her conclusion that the majority of these 'excess' orphans are consequent upon the HIV/AIDS epidemic.[12]

The initial response to this problem by policy-makers and others in Uganda and other parts of Africa was to assume that something called 'the African extended family' could cope. However, the experiences of an elderly rural couple in their eighties trying to cope with their fifteen orphaned grandchildren; of 'households' consisting only of several orphaned children all under the age of fifteen endeavouring to support themselves with occasional assistance from relatives; of apparently swelling numbers of 'street children' in Nairobi and other African towns and cities (not all but at least some of whom are AIDS orphans), has begun (but only slowly and unevenly) to persuade concerned people that 'the extended family' probably cannot cope on its own, or in some cases at all.

This raises important issues concerning the care of orphaned children: not only their physical and moral welfare, but also their educational needs and their legal protection. Among the issues is that of targeting assistance: how does one distinguish, or should one distinguish, between the needs of AIDS orphans and other equally needy orphans, or even of poor, non-orphaned children? And, related to this issue is that of institutional versus non-institutional care and the cultural specificities of such arrangements. These issues, which have been explored to some degree in Africa, are certainly of relevance to any discussion of longer-term impact in India. However, they may take on other dimensions and raise other concerns given some specific features of Indian culture and tradition.

---

12. S. Hunter: 'Orphans as a window on the AIDS epidemic in Sub-Saharan Africa: initial results and implications of a study in Uganda', *Social Science and Medicine*, Vol. 31, 681–90, 1990.

Brief discussions with a number of village people in rural Rajasthan as well as with others in urban areas suggest that there exists a degree of ambivalence about the capacity or the willingness of 'the extended family' to cope with additional members. In Paderi village, Rajasthan (the jatis represented consisting mainly of Patels, Meghwals and a few Brahmins with an Adivasi [tribal] outlier settlement), informants suggested that, under current circumstances, it was almost certain that orphans would be taken in by a paternal uncle or aunt and that, in the absence of such individuals, the wider jati would endeavour to care for the orphans, the aim being to keep the children in the family home and support them there. Given that in these communities women marry out of the village of their birth and go to live with the family of their husband, it seems likely that a widowed woman (who is not permitted to remarry) might find it particularly difficult to care for her children in the village of her husband's family, where she certainly has no rights to land, but may also find it quite difficult to move away. The situation seems particularly acute in Rajasthan, where there are five times as many widows in the population as widowers. This raises issues about both the rights of widows, the care of orphans, and, in particular, the care of female as opposed to male orphans, an important problem given the issue of the 'missing' females in the Indian population. (See the next chapter—ed.)

In extreme circumstances, the wider jati would collect money to support doubly orphaned children, but this was noted to be a rare practice. However, it was also noted that an orphan could not expect to have the same entitlements to education, welfare etc as the natural child of a household. This observation may be particularly significant in the case of female orphans who, we were told, might face serious difficulties because of the need for a dowry when they came to marry. In addition, informants seemed clear that they would not feel the same obligations to care for orphans from a jati different from their own.

Similar discussions with people in Severi village, a tribal community, elicited slightly different responses. This is also an exogamous, patrilocal community, and it was stated that in cases of both parents dying there was an equal possibility that children would go to either the male or female side of the extended family.

The conclusion of this brief discussion of the particularities of orphaning as it was observed in a few interviews in a small number of villages in Rajasthan, is that increased orphaning in India is likely to raise not only the types of issue which have been noted above from the African experience, but also perhaps some peculiarly Indian problems, some of which are already under active debate in India but which might receive an additional impetus, were greatly increased rates of orphaning to be observed in the next decade. These issues include: given the relative parallel lives of different jatis in the same spatial community, the special problems associated with the relatively limited number of local people who would be prepared to contribute to the care of a child from a jati different to their own. This assertion requires further exploration.

It is certainly the case in Africa that recognition of responsibility for orphans outside the lineage of the parents is limited, but my impression is that how 'the lineage' is practically operationalised in Africa in such circumstances may be wider than the way in which the jati is operationalised in India. Here reference may be made to the not uncontroversial article by Caldwell, Caldwell and Quiggin[13] about the African lineage and the importance of maintaining its strength and I assume on my own observations, the greater acceptability of additional children by a patrilineage than may be the case in India.

Related to the preceding comment, the treatment of female orphans is a particular issue. It may be argued that while village people state clearly that orphans cannot be expected to be treated the same as natural children with regard to material entitlements

---

13. J. Caldwell, P. Caldwell & P. Quiggin: 'The social context of AIDS in Sub-Saharan Africa', *Population and Development Review,* Vol. 15 No. 2, 185–234, June 1989.

and occupy a junior position in the household, then, in contrast to Africa, where female orphans may often be seen as an addition to the reproductive potential of the lineage, female orphans in India may be at an additional disadvantage (and even at risk) because of the looming problem of dowry as they approach marriageable age (which may of course be quite young in these communities, giving the adoptive household little enough time to raise the money even were they disposed to do so). The potential treatment of these under-dowried young women by the families of their husbands might also be considered another cause for concern.

Rural Households: Care of the Elderly

Loss of the members of the reproductive and productive cohorts of the population from any society obviously produces problems in relation to production and child care. It is often not recognised that it also presents problems in the care of the elderly. It has been suggested that in societies where there is little or no state provision for the care of the aged, their children are an insurance for the future when they become dependent. Although this problem has not been studied in detail in Africa, there is some evidence that with the loss of adult children in large numbers this safety net is removed. How important this is, is poorly understood, but a few observations and some anecdotal material suggest that among poorer elderly households, the problem may become very severe indeed. First there is the obvious loss of vitality with resulting difficulty in looking after basic needs for food and shelter, even before the illnesses and infirmities of old age become manifest. Secondly, there may be the loss of remittances from children who have moved to the cities. Thirdly, as noted previously, there may be the additional burden of orphan grandchildren—although of course, the presence of older grandchildren in a household may actually relieve some potential labour-related (but probably not cash income-related) problems.

In Indian circumstances, it seems quite likely that the situation will be very similar to that being experienced in Africa, although there are certain cultural features which may make for additional problems. The issue revolves around the differential evaluation of sons and daughters and their respective obligations. Rural families report that for reasons of pride people will not take money from their daughter's husband; this would look as though their son(s), if any, are neglecting their duty. It was reported that people were prepared to suffer some degree of hardship in order to avoid taking money from their daughters' husbands. In the event that a son dies, therefore, it must be assumed that, in addition to the emotional impact, the financial impact on the parents will also be greater than in the case of the death of a daughter. The practical implication of these observations is that the epidemic may produce an additional number of impoverished rural (as well as urban) elderly households requiring some kind of support from outside their own community.

Conclusion

On the evidence of material presented in this chapter, the situation in India differs markedly in several respects from that in Africa. In particular, while the epidemic is likely to produce, or reinforce, many of the existing problems of poverty and present them in new forms, it is less likely to have adverse effects on the subsistence agricultural sector, which appears to suffer from constraints of land and water rather than of labour.

This analysis is based on the situation in a number of rural communities in the area around Udaipur. The majority of tribal households are not solely dependent upon farming, having inadequate land for their needs and having to search for other income-earning occupations, particularly labouring work, both locally, in adjacent towns, and at greater distances. In relation to this area of India and in comparison with the 'African' situation, it does not seem conceivable that even the levels of mortality and morbidity seen in some regions of Africa could produce a general crisis of labour in these farming systems.

This having been said, in poorer and even middle-level households where the livelihood strategy depends upon income from wage work as a major component of household survival, the loss of earned income consequent upon the death or illness of a household member would, inevitably, have very distressing effects on household welfare—a general feature of any household which depends upon the labour market for its survival.

CHAPTER EIGHT

Gender Differentials and the Special Vulnerability of Women

SHAHID ASHRAF AND PETER GODWIN

Gender Differentials in Basic Statistics[1]

The sex ratio of the population over the last two decades has declined from 930 (in 1971) to 927 (in 1991) females per 1000 males. Amartya Sen has suggested that this means that some 30 million women are missing from India's population (Sen, 1991). A study in Bombay shows that as many as 40,000 female foetuses were aborted during 1984 (Joshi and Smith, 1987). There were three sex detection centres in Mumbai in 1982 as compared to twenty in 1987 (Chatterjee and Kapoor, 1990).

Life expectancy has increased for males between 1971 and 1991 from 50.5 years to 57.7 years: for females the increase has been from 49 years to 58 years. While age-specific death rates have also improved for both women and men, the differentials caused by high female mortality associated with reproduction in young adulthood remain. Interestingly, female mortality rates fall sharply, below those of men, once the reproductive age is past (Figure 1). One result of this is that there are three times as many widows in the population as widowers.

Among social indicators, while male literacy has increased from 46 per cent in 1971 to 64 per cent in 1991, female literacy has increased from 22 per cent in 1971 to only 39 per cent in 1991. Overall school enrolment is much higher for males than for

---

1. We are indebted to Dr Prateep Roy for the literature review of gender differentials he completed for us as a basis for this section.

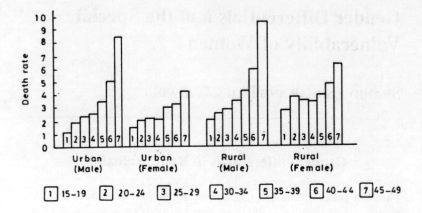

FIGURE 1: Age-specific death rates by sex and residence in India.

females. According to one study, the enrolment rates for boys and girls only equalise when per capita household expenditure reaches around Rs 225. Only approximately 5 per cent of rural and 15 per cent of urban families have an expenditure above this level.

On the utilisation of health services, a study conducted by the All India Market Information Survey in 1990 (John and Lalita, 1995), among 18,102 households and spread over 21 states and union territories, shows that female children have a lower number of medical contacts than the other members of the household. It was found that among all the children in the Paediatric Department in Ludhiana (Punjab), only 34.8 per cent were girls. Only 16.5 per cent girls were among those hospitalised and of those who died during hospitalisation, more girl children died as they were more often brought late to the hospitals, showing gross neglect on the part of the parents towards the girl child (John and Lalita, 1995).

Work participation of women as depicted in the census figures shows that the proportion of men in the labour force is more than double that of women; women, however, provide twice as much agricultural labour as men. More detailed trends in women's employment are difficult to assess owing to lack of data. Duvvury (1989) showed a decline in female employment based on 1961 and 1981 census figures. The formal sector of services and manufacturing employed only 9.6 per cent of the total labour force and 5.6 per cent of the female labour force. Women are also under-represented in the formal sector (14 per cent) while the informal sector employed 94.4 per cent of the total female workforce (John and Lalita, 1995).

Migration among females and males shows some interesting differentials. According to the 1981 census (the latest date for which detailed migration figures are available) while 20 per cent of the male population are inter-state migrants, only 10 per cent of females migrated outside their state. And of these inter-state female migrants, only 5 per cent moved for employment, while 54 per cent moved because of marriage and a further 26 per cent because the family moved. Among the male inter-state migrants, 50 per cent moved for employment, and only 24 per cent because of marriage or the family moving.

Gender Differentials: Roles, Assets and Access

Infection with HIV, and the ensuing morbidity and mortality, poses shocks and threats to households. Some of the socio-economic differentials in these shocks and threats have been identified: poor households can ill afford to lose wage-earners, and have fewer household assets to draw upon.[2] It is important, however, to understand the gender differentials in these impacts: ways in which women's status and access to assets and services affect their ability to cope with these shocks; ways in which women's roles in households determine particular patterns of household response.

---

2. David Bloom & Peter Godwin (eds.), *The Economics of HIV and AIDS: The Case of South and South East Asia,* OUP, 1997.

What are the gender differentials in these situations? Three aspects of the status of women in India provide a useful framework to analyse this: roles, assets and access. The term 'role' is used broadly to mean not only the different kinds of roles per se performed but also contributions to, and demands on household welfare that women and men make; by 'assets' is meant the differing availability and access to assets between men and women; and by access is meant the access to social, production and welfare services, including education, health care, agricultural extension, etc. While no overall assessment of these differentials, and particularly with any kind of reference to HIV has been made, a good deal of information is available.

Concerning *roles,* i. e. functions, contributions to and demands on household welfare, a good indication of the issues involved is the relationship between women's work and the health, nutrition and welfare of household members, particularly children. A World Bank Country study on India states: 'In fact, along with education, the ability to earn and control income appears to be one of the most powerful determinants of women's status in the family.'[3] The study, drawing on a number of specific micro-studies, goes on to demonstrate this connection. In an all-India study of rural households, 'Female employment was more significant than present wealth or parents' educational status in explaining variations in sex-specific survival rates. Significantly, a rise in male employment exacerbated the difference between boys' and girls' survival in favour of boys.' Further, '...whether on- or off-farm, female employment was a more important determinant of the dietary intakes of children than income or landholding size.'

As Meera Chatterjee's analysis of women's health and productivity shows, ill-health is an important cause of absenteeism from work among women. An increase in morbidity among women will affect their participation in the labour force; Chatterjee[4]

---

3. *Gender and Poverty in India,* A World Bank Country Study, 1991.
4. *Indian Women: their health and productivity,* World Bank Discussion Paper No. 109, 1990.

quotes studies showing absenteeism due to illness ranging from 6 per cent to 22 per cent of employed days; all consistently higher than for men; but in addition, in view of women's traditional nurturing and caring roles, increased morbidity among men may also reduce women's ability to earn income, as they stay at home to look after a sick husband, father, etc. A study undertaken in the slums of Hyderabad indicated that women's morbidity increased with additional workload and the fact that the hours spent on household work and child care did not reduce. The small increase in earning which they gained went largely towards medical expenses of a private doctor for their children, while they themselves went to the nearest MCH centre, ill-equipped and of little assistance (National Institute of Nutrition, 1993).

Chatterjee also quotes studies concerning overall time allocation and household work. On average, women contributed 70 per cent of total household labour time, though only 31 per cent of total income (both cash and kind). The World Bank study suggests that among the very poor, household welfare is even more dependent on women, and quotes the National Commission on Self-Employed Women and Women in the Informal Sector (1988), which found that among poor women an 'alarming number of families [survived] solely on the women's earnings (from 20 per cent to 60 per cent) in every group ... encountered.' Thus incapacitation of women due to illness, particularly recurring and debilitating illness, may well be far more significant in terms of household functioning than illness of men; particularly among the poor. Obviously, with the death of a woman the situation becomes acute, leading to the potential dissolution, or total dysfunction of the household as a unit.

Regarding *assets*, women are similarly disadvantaged. Harriss found that in Tamil Nadu men controlled market decisions related to food in 60 per cent of cases; in 15 per cent it was decided jointly; in only 25 per cent were women responsible.[5] The share

---

5. Barbara Harriss *The intra-family distribution of hunger in South Asia*, London School of Hygiene and Tropical Medicine, draft, May 1996.

of earned income for females in India is only 23 per cent (Ashraf, 1998). The Integrated Rural Development Project, for example, the largest credit-based poverty alleviation programme of the Government of India, has a target of 30 per cent female beneficiaries. In 1986/87, however, the World Bank poverty study found that only 15.9 per cent were women;[6] similarly, schemes such the National Rural Employment Programme and the Rural Landless Employment Guarantee Programme had only 17 per cent and 15 per cent respectively of female beneficiaries. Yet there is increasing evidence that women constitute well over two-thirds of the population below the poverty line.

With respect to HIV-related increases in morbidity and mortality, there is now clear evidence of the massive increase in household expenditure required (see Chapter 4 in the present volume and Bloom & Godwin, op. cit.). This work shows that disposing of assets ranks very high as a strategy for dealing with this. If women have few assets, and limited ability to dispose of them, their ability to manage this situation is equally limited.

Interestingly, different perceptions of vulnerability and risk to assets between men and women is shown in the differing assessments of the impact of chronic illness in the ILO survey of business workers in Madras, referred to in Chapter 6. While both men and women workers assessed equally the impact of chronic illness on broad measures such as loss of economic security (91 per cent and 96 per cent of men and women respectively), or the costs of medical care (96 per cent and 100 per cent respectively), women were much more likely than men to identify the creation of orphans (49 per cent of men and 98 per cent of women), loss of land and assets (58 per cent men, 79 per cent women), and reduction in remittances to family and friends (76 per cent men and 96 per cent women) as a result of illness. Men and women perceived equally the impact on their capacity to finance education (82 per cent men and 81 per cent women), but feared funeral costs differently (51 per cent men and 73 per cent women).

---

6. World Bank, 1991, op. cit.

The vulnerability of women is closely linked to the question of *access*: as Chatterjee shows, women have worse health than men: they tend to get the common communicable diseases more easily, and to suffer the consequences more quickly. '...cause-specific mortality data reveal that female mortality from the common, major diseases is consistently higher than that of males' (Chatterjee, 1990). In addition, they receive less health care. Chatterjee cites various studies showing markedly higher ratios of male to female admission to hospitals, treatment at Primary Health Centres, etc. 'A study of Primary Health Centres in Rajasthan revealed that five men received medical treatment for every woman.' Admission data from the large TB Hospital in New Delhi shows that over the ten years 1986–1995 females accounted for only 29 per cent of all admissions (see Chapter 5 in the present volume). Any increase in conditions leading to morbidity that is equally distributed amongst men and women is thus likely to increase ill-health among women more than among men. And while little is known about the sex-distribution of HIV infection in India, the epidemic is sufficiently advanced already that the rates of infection among men and women are likely to be approaching parity: a phenomenon observed around the world (Mann et al., 1996).

In the situations of gender inequality described above, there are likely to be severe gender differentials in how HIV infection affects households, and how they respond to it, both as units, and with respect to the male and female individuals within it. HIV tends to have its impact on households from a gender perspective in three ways: where a woman's household role is changed by the presence of an ill, and later dead, husband, whom she must look after and then replace (or find replacement or substitution for) as bread-winner; where she herself is ill and can no longer contribute fully to household welfare; and where the woman is dead, and the household must find a replacement or substitute for her presence. All three situations impact on a woman's employment possibilities, and thus the critical contribution she makes to household welfare. The policy implication is the importance of targeting women in affected households for emergency welfare.

The Responses of Health Services to Women

Considerable attention is being directed, both in India and worldwide, at how health services can be made more responsive to the needs of women, addressing both the socio-economic aspects of need, access, availability and permission (cf. Chatterjee, op. cit.) and the conceptual aspects of services for women as women, rather than simply as mothers or wives. At the same time, prevention programmes for HIV are being integrated with STD programmes within the framework of these expanded Reproductive Health services—a committee involving NACO and the Reproductive Health Programme within the Ministry of Health and Family Welfare is currently developing policy along these lines. The impending increases in morbidity and mortality resulting from the spread of HIV in India add singular urgency to the need for cost-effective programmatic design, and implementation in these areas, and to the inclusion of responses to the needs of women affected by the epidemic.

However, while HIV itself is often described as a sexually transmitted disease,[7] this is only true with respect to how it is transmitted. The nature of illness associated with HIV, and the kinds of responses necessary, are very different to those associated with other STDs; the infections of women with compromised immune systems do not tend to be associated with sexual or reproductive health. While health services and programmes which design HIV prevention activities within an STD and reproductive health framework may have some success, it is unclear how far such a framework will be adequate for

---

7.   Susannah Mayhew: 'Integrating MCH/FP and STD/HIV services: current debates and future directions,' in *Health Policy and Planning*, 11(4): 339–53, 1996, which describes what she calls 'the AIDS/STD pandemic'.

responses to the impact of the spread of HIV: ill-health arising as a consequence of HIV infection.

More needs to be known about the specific kinds of ill-health that will arise for women as a result of HIV, and the constraints on women accessing help for these. A major portion of it, however, is likely to arise from recurring episodes of the major communicable diseases: TB, pneumonia, gastroenteritis. And a quick glance at the basic minimum package for reproductive health suggests that women seeking treatment for these conditions will find little scope there; especially within the constraints that even the introduction of basic reproductive health faces.

Legal Issues: The Special Needs of Women

In a recent book Jayasuriya identifies four areas in which women face special legal and legislative needs with regard to the epidemic: screening; occupational hygiene and licensing; breast feeding, adoption and infant care; and abortion.[8] Screening covers a wide range of issues, but essentially refers to the risks, rights and responsibilities involved in testing for sero-status. Particular legal, ethical and human rights issues for women arise concerning testing at or before marriage, during pregnancy, during marriage (e.g. if a partner tests or is suspected to be positive), as grounds for divorce, etc.

Jayasuriya's category of occupational hygiene and licensing is essentially a euphemism for the sex industry; legal and human rights issues are involved not only for women actively engaged in commercial sex work, but also for a wide range of trafficking and other exploitative situations; refugee and migrant women, especially illegal migrants, are particularly vulnerable in this regard. In Jayasuriya's third category, a number of issues relating to children are involved; perhaps the most difficult concerning

---

8. D.C. Jayasuriya: *Health Law: International and Regional Perspectives*, Har-Anand Publs, New Delhi, 1997.

mothers' responsibilities and rights in the event of their being seropositive at the time they give birth. His fourth category, abortion, covers much the same problem.

Others have suggested additional areas in which women have special legal or human rights and needs (Grover, 1993). A much more difficult area, however, is where women suffer abuse without legal redress, in spite of the existence of legal provisions to safeguard their rights. The World Bank Country Study on Gender already extensively referred to states: 'So fundamental to the structure of Indian society is the patrilineal transmission of land that even laws mandating equal inheritance for sons and daughters are routinely and legally circumvented in wills and through reference to the special legal codes which apply to various religious groups.'

Addressing the Needs of Women

What is known about gender differentials in India suggests that a number of specific policies and programme strategies will be needed to respond to the growing needs of women affected by the epidemic. While little is known about gender differentials in the epidemiology of HIV/AIDS in India, as the epidemic deepens and spreads, more and more women will be affected, both directly and indirectly. And as this chapter has shown, gender differentials in access to, utilisation of, and benefit from health and social welfare services are so great, that any equitable response to the epidemic must specifically address the particular needs of women, and not lump all those affected in one non-gender differentiated group. Specific attention will need to be paid, for example, to female-headed households as a result of the male household head having died; households in which women are ill as a result of HIV infection; and households where the mother has died.

But a good deal more needs to be discovered, and urgently, in order to design such policies and programmes effectively. Some of the data needed are simply quantitative analyses of the epidemic; others will require socio-economic operations research:

- What are the transmission rates from husband to wife in the Indian setting, rural and urban?
- How long is the usual period between infection and the start of recurrent illness; and between illness and death in India?
- What are the likely and most common illnesses among women that will be associated with compromised immune-systems arising from HIV infection?
- What is the nature of care, for illness and debility, within households? Who will need to be targeted with assistance, support and training, for maximum benefit: the wives of infected men? mothers-in-law? daughters?
- How can health services, both public and private, respond urgently to these needs?
- How can credit and other poverty alleviation programmes be designed most effectvely to reach female-headed households?
- What kinds of legal, social and political support will be needed for female-headed households?

Finally, pehaps most distressing, will be the situation of children in affected households. The previous review has shown how important women's roles are in housholds with respect to child welfare, both in terms of direct care, and indirectly through their own economic productivity. As women devote more time to caring for ill husbands, suffer ill-health themselves, and eventually die, the children of the household will particularly suffer.

References

Ashraf, Shahid: Gender Differentials in India: A Preliminary Assessment in the Context of the HIV Epidemic, 1988 (mimeo).

Chatterjee, Meera: Indian Women: Their Health and Economic Productivity, World Bank Discussion Papers No. 109, World Bank, Washington DC, 1990.

Chatterjee, Meera and Veena Kapoor: *A Report on Women from Birth to Twenty*, Women's Developemnt Division, National Institute of Public Cooperation and Child Development, New Delhi, 1990.

Duvvury, N.: 'Women in Agriculture: A Review of the Indian Literature', *Economic and Political Weekly*, October 28, 1989.

Grover, Anand: HIV/AIDS-Related Law in India, in *Law, Ethics & HIV*, ed. Robert A. Glick, UNDP, Regional Project on H!V/AIDS, New Delhi, 1993.

John, Mary and K. Lalitha: Background Report on Gender Issues in India, Anveshi Research Centre for Women's Studies, Hyderabad; commissioned by the Overseas Development Administration, U.K., 1995.

Joshi, G.V. and D.G. Smith: 'Hi-tech Weapons in the Gender War', *South*, January, 1987.

Mann, Jonathan and Daniel Tarantola (eds.): *AIDS in the World II*, OUP, New York, 1996.

National Institute of Nutrition: Women's Work and its Impact on Child Health and Nutrition, Draft Report, Hyderabad, 1993.

Sen, Amartya: '100 Million Women are Missing', New York Times, November 5, 1991.

* * *

Discussion: The Personal Face of the Epidemic

PG: What about 'gender differentials', and women, and the things I have talked about in this chapter?

S: One of the most difficult issues surrounding the HIV positive women I have worked with is that of the 'second class treatment' meted out to them. Since HIV was first detected among female sex workers, who are already marginalised, women who are HIV positive are despised. Women who get infected are blamed for 'being loose', though the case is usually quite the opposite. This leads to one of the most destructive aspects of the epidemic—the stigmatisation of women with HIV; and it usually manifests in physical violence or severe discrimination.

PG: You documented the violence in the study you did and which we were able to publish through UNDP.[9] But what you are saying is that women who are HIV positive are in a sort of double jeopardy: in trouble because of the usual stigma of HIV, *and* because of the stigma of being a *woman* with HIV (which is usually associated with sexual promiscuity or commercialisation). I think the

---

9.   K. Sathiamoorthy & S. Solomon: 'Socio-economic realities of living with HIV', in *Socio-economic Implications of the Epidemic*, ed. Peter Godwin, UNDP, New Delhi, 1997.

situation has probably even a third layer: in trouble because of being a *woman*, and thus of lower general status, with less access to care and treatment, etc.

S: You are right. But then the second major issue that confronts a woman with HIV is that in most cases, by the time she learns of her own status, her husband is starting to fall sick (since women usually get the infection from their husbands) with HIV-related illnesses. So this young, often fairly newly-married woman, is forced to become both the breadwinner for the family as well as the care-giver for her partner. This she does foregoing her own health. This is turning out to be virtually suicidal for the HIV positive women I know.

PG: How do they cope?

S: They seem in fact to manage the situation better than men, considering the women I have known, who have gathered together the pieces and built from there. It is really very sad, Peter, that these women are stigmatised as the 'cause' of HIV transmission, and are violently blamed for it. In a society like ours, which has a heavy dose of male chauvinism, women with HIV are at the blunt end of the epidemic: they suffer society's condemnation, poverty, and violence from their partners, their in-laws, and, strangely, sometimes from their own families. Quite often, despite being on the receiving end of transmission, women have to protect their husbands from the stigma of HIV and to carry it themselves, for their husbands' sake. These women suffer severely from feelings of betrayal and inadequacy. They have the most to fear from disclosure: rejection, scapegoating and the violence they encounter is REAL.

Index

abortion, 171, 179, 180
adult illness costs, 2-3
African experience relevant to India, **150-70**:
  aspects studied: case rates, urban/rural, 150; elderly, care of, 168-9; epidemic spread, 158; girls, withdrawal from school, 160; impact on–farming systems, 160-1, 163, 164–household, 159, **164-70**–livelihood, 159–nutrition, 161; impoverishment, 169, 170; medical expenses, 160; opportunistic infections, 155; orphans, care of, 160; seroprevalence–according to community, 158–urban & rural, 150, 155, 161; susceptibility to infection, 159; transmission urban to rural, 155; vulnerability to increased morbidity & mortality, 159
  factors causing differences: cash-sex nexus, 153, 164; circumcision, 156, 158; climatic dryness, 151, 159, 160, 162-3, 164; diversity of country, 152; industrialisation, 152; irrigated land, 151; labour, 151, 159, 161, 163; migration, 150, 153-4; NGOs, 158-9; polygyny, 157, 158; poor health, 155; population density, 150, 154; poverty, 151, 157, 159; rural-urban interaction, 154-5; security, political & social, 152-3, 158; sexual-attitudes, 156-7–practices ('dry sex'), 155; STD, 155; transport routes, 152; tribal groups, 157, 162; urbanisation, 152, 154; women's status, 152
AIDS: 'case', 11, 16, 62
  'death', 11
  'orphans', 4, 6-7, 57, 59, 99, 160, 164-8–children, 4, 6-7, 57, 59, 99, 160, 164-8–elderly, 6-7, 99, 165, 168-9
  policy & programme needs: employment, 6, 146-9; health care reform, 7; poverty alleviation, 6; social development, 6; social welfare, 6-7
  & sexually transmitted diseases (STD) (*see* STD & AIDS)
AIDS in the world:
  African countries: 13 (TB), 14-15 (inc. proj.; mort.), 34 (beds), 44 (STD), 50 (circumcision),

Brihan Mumbai: **62-93** (T1, F2, F3, F4, F5, F8, F10); by age group, 65, **66-72** (T1, F2, F3, F4, F5), 73, 76-7; by cause, 65, 77, **80-7** (F8, F10), 89; by sex, 71; in teenagers, 66, 68, 72, 93; by ward, 72-3, 74-5 (F6), **81-7** (F8, F10), 89, 91, 93

India: age/sex specific, 1, 11-12, 171, 172 (F1); children, 135, 136 (F10); HIV-related, 1, 10, 14; hospitals, 129, 130-3 (F3, F5), 135-6 (F10), 137; impact on mortality statistics, 38-9 (T3); prime-age adults, 1, 10, 14, 16-17; projections, 2, 16, 32, 35, 36 (T2), 100-2 (T1); under-reporting, 13, 32-3

Thailand: 15-16, 25-6

multi-disciplinary care approach, 61

multi-partner sex activity, 140, 141

National AIDS Control Organisation (NACO), 28, 30, 33-4, 39, 41, 42, 45, 47, 52, 62, 178

National AIDS Control Programme (GOI), 5, 35

National Family Health Survey (1992-93), 1, 40

NCERT, 47

newborn, HIV transmission from mother, 40, 59

non-governmental organisations (NGO), role of, 60, 122, 158-9

nurses (India), 52, 56

opportunistic infections (cryptococcal meningitis, *diarrhoea*, fungal infection, *hepatitis*, herpes simplex, *herpes zoster*, Kaposi sarcoma, oral can-didiasis, *tuberculosis*), 77, 80, 98, 109-10, 155

'panchanama', 65

PLWHA (person/people living with HIV or AIDS), discussions with, 9, 26-7, 60-1, 124-5, 148-9, 182-3;

& discrimination, 26, 125, 148-9, 182-3

& financial problems, 124-5

problems faced by, 125

services needed, 61

socio-economic impact of death, 27

polygyny, 157

population density, 150, 154

'Positive Life', 61, 125

poverty & HIV/AIDS, 6-7, 138, 151, 154, 157, 159 (*see also* HIV/AIDS & impoverish-ment)

primary health care, rural (community health centres, primary health centres, subcentres), 17, 54-5

prime-age adult: illness, 96–households, 96–impact on productivity, 99

mortality (India), 1-2, 16-17, 96–policy implications, 3-5

prostitutes (*see* sex workers)

Rajan Babu TB Hospital, Delhi, 129-31 (F1, F2), 132 (F3)

'rationing of care', 127

rural-urban links, 154-5

Safdarjung Hospital, Delhi, 134-5, 137 (F11)

'safe' brothels, 49

safer sex, 40, 42, 46

school enrolment, 171-2

security: political, 152-3, 158